D1420622

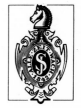

K. Hurrelmann

Human Development and Health

Springer-Verlag
Berlin Heidelberg New York
London Paris Tokyo

Prof. Dr. Klaus Hurrelmann
Universität Bielefeld
SFB 227
Postfach 8640
D-4800 Bielefeld

With 5 Figures

ISBN 3-540-50611-X Springer-Verlag Berlin Heidelberg New York
ISBN 0-387-50611-X Springer-Verlag New York Berlin Heidelberg

© Springer-Verlag Berlin Heidelberg 1989
Printed in Germany

Typesetting: Fotosatz & Design, Berchtesgaden
Printing and bookbinding: Konrad Triltsch, Graphischer Betrieb, Würzburg
2126/3130-543210 – Printed on acid-free paper

Preface

This book provides an overview of investigations into the interrelations between stressful living conditions, individual coping strategies, and social support networks, on the one hand, and physiological, psychological, and social "health", on the other. Health is used as a broad term, and is defined as a state of physical and mental well-being by which an individual is capable of processing inner and outer reality in a productive and satisfying manner. The potential stresses and strains inherent in the lifestyles of children, adolescents, and adults in contemporary industrial societies are the prime concern of this book. I try to offer a comprehensive view which takes modern socialization theory as its starting point.

Chapter 1 introduces the subject and discusses the psychological and social „costs" that accompany life within modern industrial society. *Chapter 2* reviews research on types and distribution of social, psychological, and somatic disorders. *Chapter 3* explores the risk factors and constellations of stressful life events, role conflicts, and transitions and focuses on the changes in types of demand or strains throughout the life span. *Chapter 4* contains an analysis of the personal and social „resources" that can be mobilized if stress occurs. *Chapter 5* reviews the theoretical models in sociology, psychology, and medicine; here I attempt to formulate a comprehensive socialization-theoretical model of the interdependencies between stress, development, and health/disease. *Chapter 6* discusses the potential and limits of preventive and corrective social, psychological, economic, legal, and educational interventions that serve to strengthen the personal and social resources for coping with stress.

The comprehensive view presented in this book follows modern theoretical approaches to human development that are based on the assumption that social (environmental), psychological (personal), and biological (somatic) factors jointly affect the formation of personality. The interactions between a person and his/her social environment are conceived as reciprocal interrelations. Those positions advocating a purely social determination of personality development are regarded as being just as obsolete as those that propose an organic and psychological maturation determined by natural laws. Instead,

children, adolescents, and adults are regarded as productively processing and managing external and internal reality and actively establishing and shaping relations with the organism, on the one hand, and the
societal and material environment, on the other. The concept of
development is applied to the entire life span and represents the
lifelong process of the individual's interaction with his/her living conditions. During the entire course of life, each individual faces sequential long-term changes in essential elements of personality structure
— a structure of motives, attributes, traits, attitudes, and action competences that is particular to an individual and the product of how the
individual has coped with the demands made on him/her. Successful
coping with these demands is considered to be a prerequisite of
health.

Socialization, in this book, is understood as the process of the
emergence, formation, and development of the human personality in
dependence on and in interaction with the human organism, on the
one hand, and the social and material environment, on the other.
This concept expresses the view that the human individual is permanently developing in concomitance with social and societal factors
and builds his/her personality in a process of social interaction.
According to this idea, a healthy personality does not form independently from society in any of its functions or dimensions but is continuously being shaped in a concrete, historically conveyed lifeworld
throughout the entire length of the life span (Hurrelmann 1988).

At the same time, this concept expresses the view that personality
development is subject to biological laws that are valid for all human
beings. We have to take into account a high degree of genetic determination of the individual variability in personality structures,
particulary on some levels of the physical structure and the physiological functions. The same is true for some levels of intelligence, that is,
the ability to learn and profit from experience, to adapt to a changing
environment, to motivate oneself to accomplish tasks, and to think
and reason abstractly.

Thus, the question whether human development is determined
more by the genes or more by the environment cannot be answered,
because the human organism cannot become a person except in a
social environment and can only develop in a continuous interaction
with this environment. The biogenetic vital potentials within the cellular, molecular, and organ systems influence each individual's
capacities and performance, but at the same time, any change in the
ecological and social environment has an enormous effect and acti-
vates an enormous adaptive potential on the physical, physiological,
sensory, cognitive, emotional, and social levels. The lifelong
interplay between biological, psychological, and cultural/societal
potentials and constrains determines the individual's state of health.

Starting out from this theoretical proposition, I attempt an analysis of the interaction between stress development and health.

I wish to thank Liam Gilmour, Beatrix Ahlswede, and Adelheid Baker for their careful and considerate translation of parts of this book.

K. Hurrelmann

Contents

Chapter 1 The Biopsychosocial Costs of Today's Lifestyle

Modern social systems are distinguished by their "welfare state " character. Within the framework of democratic rules, the political administration prevents extreme social inequality and provides for at least a minimum of parity in respect to the accessibility of material and nonmaterial opportunities and resources. This system functions at a tolerable level. The majority of the population within most industrial societies live in material comfort and under relatively favorable conditions. The struggle to end the mass poverty which was common up until 100 years ago has been successful in a manner which is without precedent in the history of mankind, and large sections of the population have benefited from a considerable increase in income.

Despite the relatively large successes of modern-day social systems in providing material goods and important social services, the physical, psychological, and social well-being of the population has not always been sufficiently provided for. Industrialization and urbanization have led to behavioral demands on citizens, both young and old, which are accompanied by considerable stress. In addition, industrial societies find themselves in danger of bringing forth living conditions which result in disintegration and a marginal existence among an increasing number of members of minority groups.

In this volume I address the various manifestations of social, psychological, and physiological deviance and disorders that can be interpreted, at least in part, to be symptoms of stress and deprivation. I discuss, among other things, the increase in delinquency, criminal behavior, and aggression and refer to the increase in alcoholism, drug consumption, and dependency on medication. I also discuss the growing incidence of psychological disorders and disturbances, and the rising figures for chronic diseases such as coronary disease, cancer, and psychosomatic disorders.

Many of these social, psychological, and physiological disorders which deviate from the prevailing norms can be interpreted as symptomatic reactions to "stress," as a state of biological and psychosocial tension which results from a confrontation with a variety of stress factors inherent in present-day society. I regard the aforementioned symptoms as being in part an expression of the psychosocial "costs" which accompany modern life in industrial societies. The term "lifestyle" is used here to describe the long-term organized forms and patterns of activities which take place during the process of personality development and the formation of an individual's approach to living. It expresses the manner in which an individual interacts with his/her body and the social and material environment, and defines the strategies of confronting and coping with the demands and challenges which arise during this process.

Among the variety of conditions pertaining to life in modern industrial society, the conditions of employment, that is, the structures of applying human capacities within socially organized work situations, still occupy a central position. Although, with respect to the life course, the field of employment is losing importance in a quantitative sense, and although slightly less than half of the population of industrial societes is engaged in formal structures of organized work, employment and the preparation for employment continues to dictate the standards and rules which are regarded as relevant to society in general. In particular, it sets standards which define individual performance levels and, as a consequence, individual health and well-being. As will be shown in detail, stress and conflicts in areas of work and, increasingly, within vocational and educational training which prepares for work, belong to the most obvious sources of health impairment.

The Burden of Individuality

Deviance, disorders, and diseases are often expressions of a problem being transferred from a social, societal level to psychological and physical-physiological levels. They can be indications of insoluble conflicts or inadequacy in the face of stress, both of which can very often be traced back to sociostructural conditions. At any particular point in history, the material, economic, and cultural conditions within society form parameters within which people structure their lives.

In many areas of modern-day society, a great degree of freedom exists in respect to how individuals structure their lives. Patterns of behavior are only partly determined by membership in social organizations and groups such as the family, community, religious groups, and work collectives. Usually, a person is a member of a number of structured social situations at one and the same time. He/she operates within a varied and complex social structure and is therefore forced to adapt to changing behavioral demands, to cope with conflicting value systems, and to be responsible for developing principles in controlling his/her own behavior.

The social structures of modern society are relatively open and subject to continual social change. This demands a high degree of social mobility on the part of society's members. However, it is typical of industrial societies that the behavior of their members is only partially controlled by society. Persons are only to a limited degree "absorbed" by social institutions and are therefore able to maintain a degree of freedom by which they can view themselves removed from the context of the family, religious order, community, employment situation, etc.

In a historical analysis of social systems, Norbert Elias (1987) showed clearly the freedoms and restrictions, rewards and costs which evolved in the transition from small, closely knit communities based on lineage or mutual protection, to the heterogeneous, pluralistic, present-day society. Accordingly, from a historical perspective, the potential for individuality has increased to a degree unprecedented in human history.

Elias defines individuality as the quality which directs behavior in relationships with persons and things, and as an expression of the particular style and degree by which this quality differs from that of other persons (Elias 1987, p. 87). People in modern industrial societies differ in respect to this quality of psychological processing and in their strategies of self-regulation. All of them, however, are constrained by the social and material living conditions in a way which affects all aspects of their behavior and psychological self-regulation.

This high potential for individuality is acquired at the cost of a loosening of social and cultural ties; this leads to tension and imbalance in respect to social demands of behavior and value systems, and on the psychological mechanisms of self-control. From this perspective, the road to modern society is fraught with increasing social and cultural insecurity and uncertainty in respect to the future, and to contradiction and anomy in terms of norms and values. We are experiencing a high degree of disintegration and segmentation of behavioral demands within various areas of life, which show a tendency to separate from each other and, increasingly, to organize themselves as autonomous systems. Thus, we are faced with an increasing number of alternatives and a considerable freedom of choices, each of which can, to a great extent, be dealt with by persons on an individual basis.

However, as Elias has emphasized, we not only have the potential to become more self-sufficient, we must realize this potential if we are to cope adequately with the increase in choices with which we are confronted. The possibility and the necessity of more pronounced individuality is a circumstance within social transition that everyone living in present-day society necessarily has to face (Elias 1987, p.167). The evolution of society opens up possibilities for individual development and provides new forms of satisfying and fulfilling needs. However, at the same time, modern society creates new forms of social stress and new potentials for suffering, discomfort, and uncertainty which coincide with the high degree of self-regulation required of each individual. In addition, it involves the risk of bringing forth new forms of social inequality due to the lack of equality in the way that resources for the development of action are distributed.

The principles along which modern industrial societies are organized have led to a dissolution of stages and transitional phases in the life course. The transition from one phase to another is not always clearly identifiable, and the points at which this process of transition commences and terminates are not always recognizable. For example, the transitions from childhood to adolescence, from adolescence to adulthood, and from adulthood to old age are not only shifted temporally; they also change in respect to the importance which they have for the individual. The transitions are only partially determined by the social framework; they also demand coordination and synthesis on the part of the individual. Within these areas, both the freedom of behavioral choices and the demands on the individual's self-control have increased (Kohli 1978; Beck 1986; Meyer 1986).

We must therefore conclude that within our society, despite a high standard of living, extensive services in the areas of education, child-rearing, and professional psychological counseling, social security, and a high standard of medical technology, a growing number of people are suffering from psychological or physical complaints. Evidently, economic, cultural, social, material, and ecological living conditions are so unfavorable that a large number of individuals resort to unproductive and unsuitable coping strategies. Stressful factors of a physical, psychological, social, economic, and ecological nature overtax the resources available for productively interacting with living conditions. Somatic, psychological, and social disorders must be seen as being expressions of inadequacy in processing social reality.

The Concept of Socialization

In this volume, I attempt to combine various premises and theoretical concepts which can be interpreted from the perspective of a comprehensive theory of socialization. The newer theoretical approaches in socialization research are based on the premise that physiological, psychological, and social factors have a combined influence on personality development. The relationships between the person and the environment are regarded as complex interactional processes. Moreover, the concept of socialization is used to describe the entire life span (Hurrelmann 1988, p.6):

According to my understanding, socialization is the process of the emergence, formation and development of the human personality in dependence on and in interaction with the human organism on the one hand and the social and ecological living conditions that exist at a given time within the development of a society on the other hand. Socialization designates the process in the course of which the human being with its specific biological and psychological disposition becomes a socially competent person endowed with the abilities and capacities for effective acting in the larger society and the different segments of society, and dynamically maintains this status throughout the course of his/her life.

Socialization, therefore, expresses the fact that the individual finds himself/herself in a permanent process of development that is influenced by social and societal factors inherent in social interactions. According to this view, the functions and dimensions of personality cannot develop independently of society; instead, human development takes place throughout the entire life time and within a historically determined, material and social environment (Hurrelmann & Ulich 1980; Wentworth 1980; Gecas 1981; House 1981b).

This concept of socialization appears suited to incorporating various scientific premises concerning research into relationships between stress and coping factors in the course of human development which have been elaborated within psychology, psychiatry, social medicine, social pedagogy, and sociology. It can be used to identify social, psychological, and physical factors which contribute to deviance, disorder, and disease, and to analyze personal and social resources in order to actively influence living conditions and lifestyles.

The Concept of Health

In addition to socialization, "health" is a key term in this volume. I am convinced that we have to digress from purely medical views of health. The World Health Organization introduced a definition that has attracted much attention and criticism. It defined health as "not only the absence of disease and impairment, but the state of complete physical, psychological and social well-being" (WHO 1946). This definition reflects the necessity of attempting to go beyond the narrow context of the highly professionalized health services. The enormous increases in the costs of professionalized health services within industrialized societies are in no way accompanied by an improvement in community-oriented health services or by a corresponding decline in the incidence of death and disease.

In contrast to the viewpoint prevalent in medicine, the comprehensive definition of health proclaimed here emphasizes the integration of well-being into all of the dimensions of daily life. Self-responsible behavior and self-regulation are regarded as essential factors in the development of a healthy personality. Thus, health-conscious and health-promoting lifestyles can only be expected when the prerequisites for such factors are available. Health, therefore, is both a personal and a collective variable.

Health describes the objective and subjective state of well-being that is present when the physical, psychological, and social development of a person is in harmony with her/his own possibilities, goals, and prevailing living conditions. Health is impaired when demands that arise in one or more of these areas cannot be coped with by the person in his/her respective stage of life. The impairment may be manifest in symptoms of social deviance, psychological disorder, or physical-physiological disease.

Thus, health is composed of physical, psychological, and social aspects which influence each other reciprocally. Health is closely connected to individual and collective value systems and behavior patterns which are manifest in personal lifestyles. It is a state of equilibrium which must be continuously maintained during the life course. It is not a state of well-being that is passively experienced, as suggested by the purely physical definition within classical medicine; instead, it is the result of actively pursuing the establishment and maintenance of a social, psychological, and physical capacity for action. Social, economic, ecological, and cultural living conditions thereby form the framework within which the potential for health can develop (Levi 1971, 1975; Cohen & Syme 1985; Clausen 1986a, 1987).

Thus, the definition of health used here is based on the same theoretical premises as the concept of socialization. Health is regarded as a part of the individual's development during the life course; as a process that can only take place when an individual is able to be flexible and effective in coping with internal and external demands, to achieve a satisfactory sense of continuity in experiencing him/herself, and to effect personality growth in accordance with and in consideration of the respective interaction partners. Health reflects the subjective processing of and coping with social conditions. Health is only possible when a person is able to establish constructive social relationships, is socially integrated, able to adapt his/her individual lifestyle to the changing stressful aspects of the environment and thereby secure personal self-regulation and act in accordance with the prevailing biogenetic, physiological, and physical capacities.

The following chapters take up this concept and elaborate the following propositions:

1. Social deviance, psychological disorders, and physical illness are widespread in modern Western societies. They all have to be viewed as symptoms of the overtaxing of an individual's adaptive capacities on different levels (Chapter 2).
2. Delinquency, mental illness, and physiological disorders are various manifestations of an inefficient and unproductive way of coping with external and internal demands (stressors) during the life course (Chapter 3).
3. The individual's capacity for productively coping with stressful life events, social role tensions, and biographical transitions is due to a lack of personal and social resources. The individual coping style and the social support network of an individual are the most important moderating variables in the relationship between stress, development, and health (Chapter 4).
4. Recent theoretical approaches in medicine, psychology, and sociology exhibit a convergence in their way of explaining the relationship between stressors (risk factors) occurring during the course of human development, on the one hand, and stress outcomes (symptoms), on the other. It is possible to draw together the main parts of these explanatory approaches into a socialization-theoretical model (Chapter 5).
5. Since social, psychological, and physiological disorders are the result of lifelong developmental processes, any form of intervention has to consider this fact. The most effective forms of intervention are of the preventive type, focusing on strengthening both the personal and the social resources (Chapter 6).

Chapter 2 Symptoms: Social, Psychological, and Physiological Disorders

In this chapter I approach the varieties of human behavior that do not correspond to social, psychological, and physiological norms. Within each society, whether or not a particular behavior is classified as "normal" is determined by the definition of normality prevailing within the respective society; and a question of definition is invariably a question of power. Thus, we have to ask, which persons or groups have on which legitimized basis which possibilities to classify human behavior as being socially conform, psychologically adapted, and physically healthy? And in addition, what behavioral possibilities and restrictions are connected with a person's being classified as deviant, disturbed, or unwell?

The Spectrum of Behavior Disorders

In an attempt to simplify a discussion of the social, psychological, and somatic components of human behavior, the terms "deviance" or "disorder" are used here to describe behavior that does not adhere to the standards of "normality." These terms are chosen in an attempt to remain on a descriptive level and to avoid stigmatizing.

Social Deviance

In all societies, economic and political structures, cultural traditions, and statutes and laws within the judicial system form a framework of rules which define social behavior as being "normal." Behavior which goes beyond the bounds of this framework is classified as a disorder or deviance.

Behavior of a kind which is defined as unusual and inappropriate without being perceived as sufficiently incongruent that the structure and traditions of society are challenged is referred to as nonconforming. Behavior that transgresses the boundaries of "normality" to a degree whereby it loses touch with the basis of social conformity to the extent that it provokes social tolerance is usually referred to as delinquent or criminal behavior. Such behavior is thus in conflict with cultural traditions and normative behavior as defined by law. Should this behavior be discovered, it is prosecuted and punished by the institutions of social control (police, public prosecutor, courts) on the grounds that it interferes with or prevents peaceful coexistence among the members of society (Farrington, Ohlin, & Wilson 1986).

Throughout the historical development of societies, examples can be found whereby the definition of conformity has varied in breadth. Behavior which at an earlier stage in the development of society was classified as normal, can, at a later stage, be regarded as abnormal. An example of this can be seen in the physical conflicts and acts of violence which, several generations earlier, presumably were not so intensively subject to judicial proceedings as is usually the case today. We can also observe that, during the course of history, behavior which at one time was regarded as deviant, in later times came to be accepted as normal. In this case, the level of tolerance has been raised in respect to the definition of abnormal behavior, and that section of behavior which is regarded as conformatory has increased. One example of this is given in religious or political movements which deviate from the attitudes of the majority of the population within a society. In addition, a comparison of various cultures and nations reveals great differences in the definition of abnormality (Elliot, Huizinga, & Ageton 1985).

A sensitive and comprehensive definition of social deviance has to reflect these contextual effects. Such a definition has been given by Jessor and Jessor, who define deviance as "problem behavior": It is behavior "that is socially defined as a problem, a source of concern, or as undesirable by the norms of conventional society and the institutions of adult authority, and its occurrence usually elicits some kind of social control response" (Jessor & Jessor 1977, p.33).

Following Jessor and Jessor, most of the modern definitions implicitly assume that different manifestations of deviance have a common source. For instance, social scientists have argued that strong affiliation with peer groups leads to early cigarette smoking, early sexual intercourse, marijuana use, and criminal behavior. Theorists who simultaneously address several froms of deviance within a single explanatory framework assume that various behaviors may be serving as alternative manifestations of a more general cause — for example, an alienation from the norms of conventional society and/or the absence of social bonds or the modeling and reinforcement of delinquent behavior by process of social learning. The findings of Jessor and Jessor support the possibility that shared influences create relationships between different deviant behaviors. Factors that strongly influence one deviant behavior (such as delinquency) similarly influence other behaviors (such as alcohol and drug use) (Osgood, Johnston, O'Malley, & Bachman 1988). Similarly, Dryfoos (1988, p.25) cites many studies that confirm the hypothesis that problem behaviors are, indeed, highly interrelated, and manifest different forms of deviance from and opposition to the prevailing social culture and value system:

Early initiation of sexual activity is related to the use of cigarettes and alcohol, use of marijuana and other illicit drugs, lower grades, school dropout and delinquency. ... Early initiation of smoking and alcohol leads to heavier use of cigarettes and alcohol and also leads to the use of marijuana and other illicit drugs. ... Delinquency is associated with early sexual activity, early pregnancy, substance abuse, low grades and dropout. These behaviors are interrelated, but we cannot say from this review of studies which behaviors are causes, and which are effects. One clear sense that can be derived is the impact of early initiation of any of the behaviors. Starting any one of the behaviors early appears to produce more negative outcomes and to rapidly 'spread' to other realms of behavior.

Psychological Disorders

In assessing the degree of normality in behavior from a psychological perspective, the person forms the focus of attention rather than do systems of normative social rules. Whereas the identification of social disorders serves to recognize risk factors which threaten the functioning of society as a whole, the identification of psychological disorders serves to register risks which jeopardize personality functioning and optimal personal development. A disorder exists when behavior does not correspond to prevailing developmental norms, and when its severity and duration represent a danger to further personality development.

The various forms of psychological disorders are often distinguished according to whether they are directed inwardly or outwardly. If the behavior is directed towards the social environment and contains aggressive impulses directed towards other persons, or if it expresses discontentment with social reference persons or institutions and challenges authority, it can then be referred to as exteriorizing or conflict-oriented behavior. Should the behavior be directed towards the self, contain autoaggressive impulses, or express self-deprecation or self-discontent, it can then be referred to as interiorizing or withdrawal oriented. Both types of behavior can also be found in combination (Achenbach & McConaughty 1987).

Disorders in psychological functioning are manifest in various areas of activity, for example, in relationships with other persons, in learning and achievement behavior, in adaptability, cognition, and motivation. Anxiety, social withdrawal, lack of social contacts, shyness, inhibition, depression, learned helplessness, and suicide attempts are typical forms of behavioral disorders which are inwardly directed. Behavior disorders which are outwardly directed are, for example, aggression, impulsive behavior, hyperactivity, "acting out," asocial and destructive acts.

In order to provide a standardized basis for assessing children's problems and competencies, Achenbach and his colleagues have developed a general approach that they call "empirically based assessment." They obtain reports from parents, teachers, and other reference persons via the Child Behavior Checklist (CBCL), a standardized rating scale. Examples for problem items include: can not concentrate, can not pay attention for long; is disobedient at home; gets into many fights; is unhappy, sad, or depressed. Besides the problem items, the CBCL also contains items for reporting a child's competencies in terms of the following: favorite recreational activities; jobs and chores; friends; how well the child gets along with siblings, other children, and parents; how well the child plays and works alone; school functioning.

The symptoms found through factor analysis of the Child Behavior Checklist are shown in Table 1.

The Achenbach approach supplements traditional nosologies such as the World Health Organization's *International Classification of Disease* (ICD) and the American Psychiatric Association's *Diagnostic and Statistical Manual* (DSM), which have been developed for an adult population. The Child Behavior Checklist can be used in a variety of ways: At the level of individual items, it provides a picture of the

Table 1. Syndromes found through factor analysis of the Child Behavior Checklist (from Achenbach & McConaughy 1987, p.30)

Group	Internalizing syndromes[a]	Mixed syndromes	Externalizing syndromes[a]
Both sexes aged 2–3	Social withdrawal Depressed	Sleep problems Somatic problems	Aggressive Destructive
Boys aged 4–5	Social withdrawal Depressed Immature Somatic complaints	Sex problems	Delinquent Aggressive Schizoid
Boys aged 6–11	Schizoid or anxious Depressed Uncommunicative Obsessive-compulsive Somatic complaints	Social withdrawal	Delinquent Aggressive Hyperactive
Boys aged 12–16	Somatic complaints Schizoid Uncommunicative Immature Obsessive-compulsive	Hostile withdrawal	Hyperactive Aggressive Delinquent
Girls aged 4–5	Somatic complaints Depressed Schizoid or anxious Social withdrawal	Obese	Hyperactive Sex problems Aggressive
Girls aged 6–11	Depressed Social withdrawal Somatic complaints Schizoid-obsessive		Cruel Aggressive Delinquent Sex problems Hyperactive
Girls aged 12–16	Anxious-obsessive Somatic complaints Schizoid Depressed withdrawal	Immature Hyperactive	Cruel Aggressive Delinquent

[a] Syndromes are listed in descending order of their loadings on the second-order Internalizing and Externalizing factors

specific problems and competencies reported for a child; at the level of total problem scores, it provides a summary index of deviance from norms for the child's age and sex; and at the level of the profile pattern it offers a taxonomy of behavior disorders.

Those psychological abnormalities that are long-lasting and strongly connected to the personality structure can be classified as psychiatric disorders. Following the definitions of Murphy and Leighton (1965, p.12), we can define psychiatric disorders as those behaviors, emotions, attitudes, and beliefs commonly regarded as warranting psychiatric help. More specifically, the term includes brain syndromes, mental deficiency, the functional psychoses, psychophysiological disorders, psychoneuroses, personality trait disturbances, sociopathic behavior, and acute situational reactions. In this use, "psychiatric disorder" has a somewhat broader connotation than "mental illness," a term which is often restricted to the functional psychoses and severe psychoneuroses. It is important to note that all of these patterns of psychiatric disorder are regarded as process phenomena having an origin, course, and outcome which can be fully understood only in relation to the total life history of the individual (Dohrenwend 1975; Brown & Harris 1978; Katschnig 1981; Leavy 1983).

Obviously, in different countries with different cultural traditions, different kinds of behavior are considered normal or abnormal. This does not mean that we are completely lacking in valid standards of psychological functioning. There is evidence that some disorders are so debilitating as to gain recognition in any society no matter what its cultural patterns. It is apparent that tendencies toward these symptoms can be part of a person's genetic and constitutional heritage and may be precipitated, maintained, or inhibited by such physiological events as a long illness or sustained malnutrition. On the other hand, the functioning of persons with psychiatric disorders which are chiefly of hereditary or physiological origin may relate significantly to their sociocultural setting. Any definition of psychological or psychiatric disorder has to be sufficiently broad in order to include various types of reactions to life stress or malfunctions (Simmons 1981).

It is important to note that psychological problem behavior can be distinguished from normal behavior only gradually. We have to emphasize that the cutting points between types of behavior are not clearly identifiable and are dependent on many singular factors (Gurland 1976). There exist no generally accepted professional concepts and terms that describe and classify problem behavior. As a result, socially legitimated help- and prevention-oriented groups and institutions, and the professional staff of these institutions, have a decisive influence on the practice of classification. The procedures and methods of psychiatrical exploration and the psychological tests and observations forming the basis of diagnosis are reliable only to a certain degree. The standards and categories of identifying problem behavior are still subject to much discussion among therapists.

For this reason cultural comparisons, especially comparative epidemiology, can be important scientific tools in gaining knowledge of the prevalence and incidence of disorders:

In cross-cultural studies we are at the edge of a virtually unknown continent; and hence there is a primary need for observation and information collecting. Epidemiology is one systematic way of doing this. If done successfully, it will lay a quantitative baseline from which all manner of other studies can be carried out, for it deals with one of the first questions that has to be asked in comparing psychiatric disorder in two or more cultures, more or less regardless of what the ultimate aim may be. (Murphy & Leighton 1965, p.197)

Physiological Disorders

The point of focus in the area of nonnormal physical and physiological behavior is the proper functioning of the human organism. All disorders that deviate extensively from the state of normality in terms of intensity, frequency, and duration can be classified as organic, physical, or somatic disorders. According to this view, impairments of the normal physiological functions are understood as the organism's inability to adapt to and cope with specific internal and external demands. As in the case of social and psychological normality, organic normality has also to be understood as a state defined by certain standards. A digression from normality takes place if the body's immune system is weakened to the extent that it is unable to resist factors which lead to illness and disease, or if the person's psychological and health-related social behavior results in inappropriate reactions to bodily demands (Matarazzo, Weiss, Herd, Miller, & Weiss 1984).

Symptoms of organic impairment are, for the most part, classified according to the cause of disease, which can ensue either from:

1. Microbiological agents such as viruses or bacteria which lead to various infectious diseases ("acute diseases"), such as tuberculosis or measles, or
2. Prolonged taxing of the physical, psychological, or social adaptability, which leads to chronic illness such as cardiovascular disease and cancer

Despite the great variety of causal factors, common sources can be recognized that lead to both groups of organic impairment. They are found in the overtaxing of the social, psychological, and biological capabilities of adaptation that can influence each other and can then form the point of departure for the emergence and development of a disease. Both acute and chronic diseases make great demands on the organism's regulatory capacity, which is overtaxed if the immune system is unable to control the spread of an infectious disease or cell growth. Overloadings that initially occur on the physical level can gradually find expression in the psychosocial and social behavior of a person (Levi 1971, 1975). This is shown by the fact that psychological and physiological disorders frequently overlap, especially among patients with chronic illness such as high blood pressure, coronary heart condition, insomnia, asthma, and stomach ulcer. Many of these illnesses become chronic due to a psychodynamic overlapping or as a result of reactions from the environment (Petermann, Noecker, & Bode 1987, p.29).

A positive relationship between physical illness and psychological distress has been consistently reported. For example, Langner and Michael (1963), as well as Aneshensel and Fredrichs (1982), have shown that physical illness is a cause of depression. Turner and Noh (1988), in their study, report evidence for the fact that physically disabled persons find it especially difficult to achieve and maintain psychological well-being. On the basis of data obtained from a large representative sample of physically disabled subjects, the authors present evidence confirming the hypothesis that the physically disabled are at dramatically increased risk of suffering from symptoms of depression. Although the extent of increased risk appears to be slightly higher among men than among women, and somewhat greater for those 65 years and older than for younger subjects, the results indicate that physical disability is associated with significantly increased risk for depression, regardless of gender or age (Turner & Noh 1988, p.34).

Whereas within the area of infectious, "acute" diseases the connection to social and psychological capabilities of adaptation is still under discussion, the social and psychological implications of noninfectious "chronic" diseases have been proved frequently over the past years (Corson & Corson 1983; Dillon, Minchoff, & Baker, 1985; Kaplan 1985). Elliot and Eisdorfer (1982), in their overview report, sum up the evidence for the effects of social and psychological stress on various types of chronic diseases:

1. Cardiovascular diseases: In the case of artherosclerosis, for example, which refers to the accumulation of large plaques of lipids in the major arteries, thereby cutting off the blood supply to such vital organs as the heart and leading to angina and myocardial infarction, a relationship was found with aggressive and competetive personality characteristics and acute and chronic social and psychological stressors. Similar statements can be made for cardiac disturbance and high blood pressure. The ability of acute stressors to aggravate heart failure through increased work load also has been well documented. In most cases, reactions to stressors interact with preexisting cardiac pathology. Bereavement, loss of prestige, and loss of employment have all been implicated as risk factors for myocardial infarctions. Sociocultural changes such as major changes in living arrangements or occupation and discrepancies between the culture of origin and the current cultural milieu also significantly increase heart-attack risk.
2. Cancerous diseases: Here also, increasing evidence was found that points to a relationship with personality factors, familial constellations, particular coping strategies, and social living conditions, including several lifestyle variables.
3. Gastrointestinal diseases: Here — especially in the case of stomach ulcers — a relationship was found with living and working conditions that put strain on the sociopsychological capacity for adaptation. For example, emotional states can influence stomach acid secretion — anger and hostility increase it, depression and withdrawal decrease it.
4. These relationships also apply in the case of pulmonary diseases, especially bronchial asthma, skin diseases, and allergies.

The immunological systems of the body seems to be closely connected with other physiological processes. Social and psychological strain can impair this system's protective function in a manner that is not yet completely understood. Elliot and Eisdorfer suggest a framework for identifying important areas of stress research and point to the deficits in this research tradition. The significant areas are: Potential activators (x), reactions (y), consequences (z), and mediators:

The first area relates to identification of environmental events, or stressors, themselves and to their measurement and interrelationships; the second area comprises the delineation of the physiological, biochemical, and psychosocial processes that these stressors induce in the individual; the third entails assessment of ensuing health changes or disease consequences; and the last involves discovery of specific factors that modify interactions among the other three. Most available research demonstrates either that x and z are associated or that x can produce y. There is little or no information on how y leads to z or on important x–y or y–z mediators. (Elliot & Eisdorfer 1982, p.318)

It can be assumed that there are no specific "stress diseases" that are — to take an example — caused exclusively by social stressors (role strain, marital disharmony, unemployment, etc.). However, many research findings suggest that stress can increase the susceptibility to disease due to a decrease in resistance, insufficient opportunity for reconvalescence, and inaproppriate coping strategies, and thus accelerate, aggravate, and prolong illness whose origin is not related to stress factors (Hotaling, Atwell, & Linsky 1978; Chiriboga & Cutler 1980; Nitsch 1981, p.35; Johnson 1986).

In addition, we have to consider diseases resulting from behavior that is deleterious to physical health. This refers, for example, to excessive and uncontrolled consumption of alcohol and tobacco, as well as to the consumption of illegal substances and the abuse of medicinal and pharmacological substances. This behavior, for the most part, can be traced back to social and psychological factors, but after a certain time it can have a direct effect on physical well-being, especially as a result of the ensuing addiction (Bachman, Johnston, & O'Malley 1981; Silbereisen, Eyferth, & Rudinger 1986; Wills 1987).

The long-term consequences of chronic diseases can result in various forms of disablement and organic impairments. They, too, can be the result of accidents or genetic defects or injuries sustained during birth. The most common classification in this area is made according to whether the disorder is (a) a physical handicap (e.g., disorders of the muscles, skeleton, inner organs, central nervous system, metabolic functions), or (b) a disorder of the sensory systems (e.g., impairment of vision, hearing, speech), or (c) a deficit in intelligence (e.g., learning disability, mental retardation) (Antonovsky 1979; Haggerty 1983; Butler & Corner 1984).

To repeat, all types of disorders that have been discussed, social and psychological as well as physiological, are forms of "nonnormality" that are related to the economic, cultural, and ecological living conditions of present-day industrial societies. Within these areas, it is not always possible to distinguish between normal and abnormal behavior; rather, the dividing lines are permeable and not easily recognizable.

Which behavior is regarded as not being in accordance with normality, and what is regarded as a social, psychological, or somatic disorder depends essentially on the definitions used by the social institutions that provide assistance and assert authority and control. Whether a person's behavior appears problematic or disturbing to parents, teachers, work colleagues, street workers, psychologists, doctors, and other instances of control and provision depends essentially on the values, attitudes, and relevant capabilities for assessment and judgement. For example, parents and teachers very often differ in their estimation of what can be regarded as psychological problem behavior in youth, due to the fact that they are affected differently by the adolescent's behavior. As a result of their training in making judgements, and due to their role as representatives of an institution, social workers, psychologists, medical doctors, and psychiatrists tend to classify behavior as disorderly more quickly than do "laymen" (Rutter 1980, p.235).

In analogy, within scientific research, a definition of behavior disorder can be traced back to the respective definition put forward by the research team. The survey team's disciplinary and epistemological interests and the institutional background of the research project also play a decisive role. This explains why available surveys often differ greatly in their statements on deviant behavior and its distribution. Because the borders between deviant and "normal" behavior are permeable, the research teams mark specific, well-founded points that characterize the degree, duration, and intensity of deviance from normality that a behavior shows. This process has the advantage of not being based on a dogmatic conception of disorders. It is based on the theoretical premise that within a wide spectrum of behavior, social, psychological, and physical disorders can occur which are in need of special attention because they could have an impairing effect on further individual development.

Epidemiological Data

The following examples introduce some distributional data of selected symptoms in the areas of

1. Social deviance
2. Psychological disorders
3. Physical diseases

The data are taken from the records of several service institutions, from census data, and from scientific survey studies. We use the common epidemiological code values: The *prevalence* indicates the frequency of the symptom's occurrence (e.g., criminal behavior, attempted suicide, drug abuse, etc.) in a specified age group at a certain point in time. We make a distinction between prevalence in the life course (how often the symptom occurred up to the present) and prevalence during a particular period of time (how often it occurred in the past year, month, etc.). The *incidence* provides information on how many new cases of a symptom occurred within a certain period of time. Both values are usually oriented towards an index, for example, to 100000 persons of the respective age group.

Epidemiology of Socially Deviant Behavior

The identification of socially deviant behavior is dependent on historical and cultural traditions. In all Western industrial nations, especially among the adolescent population, changes in values and in patterns aimed at leading a meaningful life can be observed which sometimes are regarded as deviations from traditionally expected behavior. Some studies show that, among adolescents, traditional middle-class values such as the accumulation of wealth, industriousness, the acquisition of property, and social prestige become less important, whereas self-growth, sensitive lifestyle, and affectionate relationships with other people become increasingly important. Compared with former generations, changes have taken place in respect to priorities and in respect to the emphasis placed on personal and community-oriented goals. However, none of the serious studies in this area show a revolutionary change in the values of the younger generation which could disrupt social consensus. Traditional concepts of life are questioned, but a common and unified alternative lifestyle of an opposing cultural character is found only among adolescent fringe groups (Baethge 1989).

In the area of delinquent and criminal behavior, official police and court statistics on criminality and convictions can only provide rough estimates. Self-report studies show that the number of people who have committed delinquent acts far exceeds the number of people taken to court. The official statistics refer to the number of convictions each year, and not to the number of separate individuals convicted. As a result, any changes in rates of recidivism will affect the crime statistics. For these and other reasons, crime statistics provide a rather uncertain guide as to whether changes apply to levels of delinquency or to numbers of delinquents (Farrington, Ohlin, & Wilson 1986).

Scientific random sample surveys point to the fact that the real (true) prevalence of some delicts is twice as high, or higher, than the registered prevalence. These numbers are specially high among minor offenses such as using public transport without paying, driving without a license, or shoplifting. However, as Rutter shows, the official data are not without use: Self-reported delinquency (especially severe and repeated delinquency) shows substantial, though less than perfect, level of agreement with administrative figures. Thus, we can read epidemiological trends from these data:

From 1900 until the beginning of the First World War the crime rate remained fairly stable; during the next 15 years it rose about 5 per cent per annum; it then fluctuated but remained roughly stable until 1954; then during the next decade crime increased at the record rate of about 10 per cent per annum. Since 1965 the crime rate has continued to increase but at a more variable and, in general, somewhat slower rate. (Rutter 1980, p.119)

As the studies by Rutter demonstrate, delinquency rates have to be viewed against the background of historical trends in crime as a whole. In fact, it is clear that all of these trends are more evident in juveniles than they are in adults. The increase in crime rates among 14- to 17-year-old males (and also 18- to 21-year-olds) during the last two decades has been rather greater than that in adult men. Thus, crime statistics clearly show that rates of delinquency in this specific life phase have increased considerably throughout this century and especially since the Second World War.

To illustrate this tendency, let us take a closer look at the examples provided by official statistics on crime prosecution and convictions in the Federal Republic of Germany (FRG). These statistics agree on the relatively high distribution data of delinquent behavior in adolescence. According to police records, the proportion of children and adolescents under the minimal age for criminal prosecution who are

Table 2. Ratio of suspects to total population in the Federal Republic of Germany (Heinz 1985, p.63)

Age groups	Suspects (%)	Population (%)
Children (8 to 14 years)	5.6	9.1
Adolescents (14 to 18 years)	15.2	7.5
Adolescents (18 to 21 years)	13.9	5.4
Young adults (21 to 25 years)	13.4	6.6
Adults (25 years and older)	51.9	71.4
Total	100.0	100.0

suspected of crimes is much greater than their proportion of the general population (see Table 2).

As the statistics show, 42.5% of the suspects under investigation belonged to the adolescent or young adult age group (14- to 25-year-olds), despite the fact that their share of the population in the same year was only 19.5%. A similar picture emerges when comparing the percentage of adolescent convictions with their percentage of the entire population: Almost 44% of the criminal convictions related to adolescents or young adults, whereas about 50% related to adults in the same year.

Moreover, the analysis shows that since 1956 the crime rate of adolescents in the FRG has increased more than the crime rate of adults and by now far exceeds it. The highest rate is among the 18- to 21-year-olds. The rate for children is (still) the smallest, but it has drawn closer to the rate for adults. The overall increase in rates for persons registered as suspect by the police among children, adolescents, and young adults between 1963 and 1981 was 90%, for adults 37%. The number of convictions of young adults and adolescents is three times higher than that of adults. Adolescents show the largest increase, with 137% more convictions between 1954 and 1981. In contrast, the number of adult convictions in 1981 was lower than the figure for 1954 (Heinz 1985, p.65).

Studies from other countries support these results (Rutter 1980, p.120; Hirschi & Gottfredson 1983; Rutter & Giller 1983; Elliot, Huizinga, & Ageton 1985; Farrington, Ohlin, & Wilson 1986). As these figures clearly demonstrate, criminal statistics of the police and the courts show the same tendency of relatively high criminal activity among young people. However, the comparison also demonstrates that the number of suspects is several times higher than the number of persons actually convicted and that the differences between the number of persons convicted within various age groups are much smaller than the differences between the respective figures for suspects. At all events, the figures for convictions put the police statistics in perspective, the latter being heavily influenced by increasing readiness to report crimes, and increasing success in registering and solving crimes.

Further reservations arise concerning the accuracy of the statistical data if we differentiate between various groups of offenders. The above-mentioned data on crime are based on average values that do not differentiate between different developments and do not take the seriousness of the offense into account. By dividing the number of persons convicted into categories according to the type of offense, it becomes obvious that the increases in the number of convictions among adolescents and young adults result mainly from violations of traffic laws and offenses against property.

All data clearly indicate that juvenile delinquency remains relatively sporadic when viewed within the entire life course. The increase in juvenile crime does not continue into adulthood. Moreover, the prevalence of delinquent and criminal behavior differs greatly according to gender. Despite a significant increase in the figures for crimes and convictions over the past two decades, the prevalence among female adolescents and women in the FRG is still only about one-seventh of that of men. Theft in department stores and shops make up the greatest number of offenses committed by females. The number of women and female adolescents convicted of violent offenses, traffic offenses, and crimes committed in groups is extremely low in comparison (Heinz 1985, p.67).

Distribution of Psychological Problem Behavior

In order to obtain data on the distribution of psychological behavior disorders, we can refer to reports on treated prevalence, that is, to statistics on referrals to and stays in clinics and counseling centers. These reports, of course, can only record a small part of the true prevalence, because they only list extremely serious cases and, incidently, reflect selection effects that automatically occur through referrals or stays in institutions. The true prevalence marks the total proportion of persons with psychological behavior disorders within a population, including those cases that have not yet been treated or registered. In general, the figures for treated prevalence can only offer a limited assessment of the extent of true prevalence.

Psychological problem behavior shows different manifestations over the life course (Cullinan, Epstein, & Lloyd 1983). In considering treated prevalence in childhood and adolescence we find that school-related learning difficulties and achievement disorders predominate. These results indicate that the system of classifying abnormal behavior is to a large extent dependent on institutional guidelines: Parents ask for the help of advisory services if scholastic problems arise, whereas they are much more reserved if disorders in other areas occur. Additionally, the role played by social institutions in the manifestation of achievement disorders is emphasized by the fact that they are defined as the failure to meet the standards set by teachers in a particular subject within a particular school year (Hurrelmann 1987b).

Failure to meet scholastic demands has become a serious symptom of problem behavior in most industrial societies. It is most clearly documented during the transition between stages in the course of education: that is, when entering school, at the transition from elementary to secondary school, from one term to the next, and from one school type to another. In most school systems, such failures are expressed most dramatically when school-leaving certificates are allocated. In the

FRG, for example, we have to expect that an average of about 9% of each age group will not achieve the basic school-leaving diploma. Other school systems have their own definition of scholastic failure and, on completion of school, they likewise document this by withholding a high school diploma. For example, in the USA, the corresponding quota for under 20-year-olds is approximately 15% of each school year (Rumberger 1987).

In addition to learning and achievement disorders, difficulties in making social contacts and in adaptability, aggression, and suicide attempts, show the highest rates of treated prevalence in childhood and adolescence (Butler & Corner 1984). In adulthood, the more serious disorders schizophrenia, neurosis, psychosis, and suicidal acts are most prevalent (Dohrenwend 1975; Srole, Langner, Michael, Opler, & Rennie 1962; Berkman & Breslow 1983).

Representative studies which are not restricted to clinic populations and which show the "true prevalence," indicate that an average of 10% to 12% of all primary school children suffer from serious psychological disorders that are in need of treatment. In the well-known Isle of Wight study a total population of over 2000 14- to 15-year-olds was screened using parents' and teachers' questionnaires of known reliability and validity. Those with high scores (indicating the possibility of disorder), together with a randomly selected control group, were psychiatrically assessed in detail by means of interviews with parents, teachers, and the adolescents themselves. Psychiatric assessments were also available on 10-year-old children and on the parents of the adolescents, so that it was possible to examine age differences in prevalence. When the results were compared, it appeared that the overall frequency of psychological disorders was slightly higher in adolescence than in childhood and in adult life.

Putting all the information together, the one year period prevalence of disorder was probably about 10- to 15-per cent for the 14- to 15-year age group. But, in addition to adolescents with generally recognizable psychiatric disorders, there was a further group of teenagers who reported marked suffering associated with psychiatric symptomatology but whose problems were not evident to parents and teachers. When these were included, the prevalence rate rose to about 21 per cent. The clinical significance of this affective disturbance suffered by the adolescents but not obvious to others remains uncertain, but it was this phenomenon which was most characteristically different about the adolescent age period. The tentative conclusions from all the available epidemiological findings are that the great majority of adolescents are free of psychiatric disturbance but that disorders may be somewhat more frequent during the teens than during childhood, and possibly slightly more than during the middle adult life. (Rutter 1980, p.477)

The Isle of Wight study provides findings on the various types of psychiatric disorder manifest during adolescence. About two-fiths of adolescents with a psychiatric condition showed some form of emotional disorder. Most of these consisted of anxiety states, depression, or some kind of affective disorder. Obsessive-compulsive conditions, hysteria, circumscribed phobic states, and tics all affected a few individuals but were much less common. Conduct disorders occurred in about the same proportion — two-fifths of those with a psychiatric disability. A substantial minority of teenagers, about one-fifth, had disorders involving a mixture of antisocial behavior and emotional disturbance (Rutter 1980, p.48).

Many types of abnormal behavior are definitely a result of developmental stages and are of a temporary nature. They change in accordance with age and certain stages in the life course that are connected to central transitional problems. For example, hypermotoric behavior can be regarded as a childhood phenomenon, and suicide attempts are closely related to adolescence.

Taking this into account, statements on behavioral disorders in an early life phase can not simply be extrapolated to later life phases. The psychiatric disorders which do arise for the first time during adolescence differ in some important respects from those beginning in earlier childhood. Most obviously they are not associated with educational retardation in the way that is characteristic of the disorders of the prepubescent period (Rutter 1980, p.237). Only from the end of the twentieth year of life onwards can stabilizing behavioral patterns be expected. In the third life decade behavioral disorders that occur once are usually of longer duration than they would have been had they occurred earlier (Dohrenwend, Dohrenwend, Gould, Link, Neugebauer & Wunsch-Hitzig 1980).

As further demonstrated by survey studies, the gender-specific distribution of psychological disorders is characterized by an overrepresentation of males during childhood, and by an overrepresentation of females during old age. During adolescence and in early adulthood, the prevalence rates are evenly balanced. These trends were found among clinical and representative samples. They reflect the growing importance of psychological and emotional conflicts of women approaching old age. In considering symptoms like depression, neuroticism, and hysteria, we can observe, for example, how these symptoms which previously had been typical of males, become symptoms typical of females at the "turning-point" in adolescence and early adulthood (Gove & Tudor 1973; Rutter 1980, p.59). Most studies that focus on treated prevalance come to the same trend results:

> Taken together, these findings suggest a process by which two major trends occur from childhood to adolescence and from adolescence to adulthood. First, higher relative morbidity patterns among male children decline gradually through maturation into adulthood, whereas relative morbidity for females increases during this process. The second trend suggested by these studies, ... is higher rates of mental health intervention for males than for females, which decline through early adolescence into later adolescence. It has yet to be determined whether this second trend reflects accurately the higher relative morbidity patterns or (alternatively) differential rates of help seeking based on contributing factors other than morbidity. (Johnson & Kaplan 1988, p.54)

Not only are the sex differences in the overall rates of psychological disorders important — it is interesting to consider the types of psychopathology overrepresented in males or in females as well. A considerable amount of epidemiological evidence suggests than women in all age groups are more likely than men to be treated for cases of what can be labeled as intropunitive problems, namely, disorders resulting from the internalization of conflict. Disorders such as depression would belong to this set of problems. In contrast, males are more likely to be treated for extropunitive difficulties in which they "act out" the conflict (for example, antisocial and paranoid personality disorders). Depression, phobia, and personality disorders are diagnosed more commonly for women, whereas personality disorders and antisocial personality disorders are more likely to be assigned to men (Gove 1985; Johnson & Kaplan 1988).

Among those psychiatric disorders that are extremely typical for girls are anorexia nervosa and bulimia nervosa. The incidence of anorexia nervosa has increased in the past 30 years both in the United States and in Western Europe (Butler & Corner 1984). Age of onset is most common between 12 and 30 and occurs predominantly in the white population. Anorexia nervosa occurs predominantly in females; most surveys report only 6% of males. Bulimia nervosa emerged only in 1980 as a distinct diagnostic entity. The prevalence of males in the bulimia nervosa population probably varies between 10% and 15%.

In the area of attempted suicide and suicidal acts, which have increased over the past years, we, too, are confronted with a particular gender-specific distribution pattern: The statistics on the prevalence of attempted suicide show that the proportion of female adolescents and women is significantly higher. On the contrary, the proportion of male adolescents and men is significantly higher for enacted suicide (Diekstra & Hawton 1986).

In all Western industrial countries the relative importance of committed suicide for adolescents in mortality statistics has increased over the past three decades, and by now stands at fourth place behind traffic accidents, homicide, and chronic diseases (Hawton 1986). Committed suicide is therefore no longer a symptom typical for old age as analyzed by Durkheim (1951) but is typical for all age groups. The relative importance of this cause of death is highest in adolescence in comparison with other life phases. Following new investigations, a significant shifting of the frequency of suicide over the life span can be observed. Berman (1986) has compiled the available statistical reports of 1960 and 1980 documenting a noticeable increase of the suicide death rate among 10- to 30-year-olds, whereas in the same period a decline of the corresponding death rate among the 30- to 80-year-olds can be observed. In comparison with the most frequent cause of death (traffic accidents), the proportions have altered. Whereas in 1960 the death rate because of suicide was at one-tenth of the rate of death because of a traffic accident, it was at one-fifth in 1980.

Physical Disorders

Within the last century, there has been a dramatic decrease in the incidence of acute, infectious diseases that were common in earlier times. The enormous successes in controlling infectious diseases by improving medical technology and hygienic conditions resulted in a substantial increase in the life expectancy of all groups of the population. The dramatic reduction in the figures for death from disease within the last 100 years can mainly be traced back to the decline in those diseases that are caused and transmitted by microorganisms (tuberculosis, chickenpox, syphilis, measles, gonorrhea, hepatitis, salmonellosis). The decrease in these infectious diseases has, however, been counterbalanced by the increase in car-

Table 3. Mortality statistics on the causes of death per 100.000 persons (for 1985)

	FRG	GB	USA	Japan
Cardiovascular diseases (all)	576	560	421	249
– Hypertension	18	9	14	11
– Myocardial infarction	132	210	122	25
– Cerebrovascular diseases	152	144	67	117
Malignant neoplasms (all)	260	278	189	153
– Stomach	25	21	6	42
– Intestines	26	23	20	9
– Rectum	12	12	4	7
– Trachea, bronchial tube, lungs	42	72	49	23
– Female mammary gland	41	52	32	8
– Prostate	28	26	22	4
Bronchitis, emphysema, asthma	36	32	9	11
Pneumonia	27	50	23	33
Liver diseases	24	5	12	14
Suicide and autoaggression	21	9	12	20
Diabetes mellitus	18	13	16	8
Traffic accidents	16	10	19	10
Infectious and parasitic diseases	7	5	9	10
Psychiatric diseases	7	22	7	3
Stomach and duodenal ulcer	5	9	3	4

Source: (Bundesministerium für Jugend, Familie und Gesundheit 1987, p. 192)

diovascular diseases, cancer diseases, and other chronic illnesses (Antonovsky 1979, p.16–25).

Official statistics on the causes of death in the different industrial countries (Table 3) show the highest number of deaths to be attributable to cardiovascular diseases (in the FRG more than 50% of all deaths), followed by cancer and diseases of the respiratory organs; infectious diseases account for only 1%.

These results are supported by medical self-reports taken from representative surveys. According to these reports, diseases of the cardiovascular system, the respiratory organs, as well as diseases of the skeletal system, muscles, and tissue are most widespread and account for 60% of all reported diseases (Waller 1985, p.53). According to the statistics, the proportion of women who report disease (17%) is significantly higher than that of men (14%).

As has already been said, many studies give evidence that we have to consider links between physiological and psychological disorders (Bräutigam & Christian 1986). The impairments that a physically ill person is exposed to affect his/her psychosocial state and, as can be proved, lead to higher quotas of psychological and social behavior disorders. These disorders are often formed during the course of chronic diseases. Generally, the more serious the physiological disorder, the more pronounced is the extent of psychological disorders. The psychological stability of a person is especially strained in cases where a disease is progressive and leads or threatens to lead to disablement (Felton, Revenson, & Hinrichsen 1984).

In all industrial societies, the proportion of people officially registered as disabled is rising. In considering physical and physiological disabilities (handicaps), we are dependent on definitions based on official diagnostic procedures in order to assess claims for rehabilitation benefits (professional re-education, tax benefits, supplementary pensions, special schooling, etc.). According to these statistics, we can assume, for example, that 14% of the total population of the FRG are disabled.

The highest proportion of handicaps (35%) result form impairments in the function of the inner organs, whereby heart and cardiac disease are reported most frequently. Disablement relating to functional disorders of the limbs, spinal column, torso, and deformation of the thorax take second place (30%). They are followed by disablements of the brain and nervous system such as paralysis, paraplegia, multiple sclerosis, epilepsy, and other impairments of this kind. In respect to impairments of the senses, official school registrations offer reliable figures. According to recent FRG statistics, the proportions of persons suffering from various defects are as follows: visual impairments or complete blindness, 0.06%; hearing impairments, 0.14%; speech defects, 0.27%; mental handicap, 0.63%; physical handicap, 0.24% (Bleidick 1987, p.68).

Among the more specific psychophysiological symptoms we include "drug addiction." Here we refer mainly to persons having a pathological relationship to a psychotropic substance, which is marked by psychological and physical dependency and a lack of control in respect to consumption of the substance. The substance is a "drug" that effects the psychological and psychosomatic well-being. For a certain period, the consumer experiences a pleasant emotional state by using legal and illegal drugs. Substances such as alcohol, nicotine, opium, and psychopharmaceuticals are consumed in order to induce an elevated mood and to avoid feelings of discomfort; they influence a person's subjective sense of well-being by acting directly through the central nervous system. The long-term effects, however, are detrimental to health; the person behaves at the expense of his own biopsychosocial system (Jessor & Jessor 1977; Kandel 1980).

In addition, we can also identify addictions that are not connected to a chemical or natural substance: for example, extreme forms of human behavior that are chosen in order to provoke feelings of pleasure or to avoid unpleasant feelings. In recent years, socially isolated and pathological behavior in connection with slot machines, video games, and extensive viewing of television has been a subject of special attention.

The introduction to substance abuse usually begins with the consumption of legal drugs during childhood — in particular, alcohol and nicotine. The majority of all adolescents restrict their drug consumption to such legal substances. A minority also experiment with "soft" illegal drugs over a period of a few years, above all, with marijuana. A small percentage of those who consume marijuana also use "hard" illegal drugs like heroin for a limited for unlimited period. The seemingly harmless legal drugs have to be regarded as a sort of forerunner of the illegal drugs. In general, first experiences are made with the drug nicotine, followed by

alcohol, marijuana, glue sniffing, hallucinogens, amphetamines, opiom deriva-
tives, tranquilizers, and cocaine (Kandel, Kessler, & Margulies 1978).

As US studies show, alcohol use rose during the late 1970s. The large majority
of high school seniors (two-thirds of the females and more than tree-fourths of the
males) reported some use during the month prior to questioning. The most serious
drinking problem among adolescents is reflected in a different item: when asked
how often they had taken five or more drinks in a row during the prior 2 weeks,
52% of the males and 31% of the females reported doing so on at least one occa-
sion (Bachman, Johnston, & O'Malley 1981, p.60).

Tobacco consumption, according to the same study, is also widespread among
adolescents. At the end of the second lite-uecade the figures approximate those of
the total adult population. According to relevant surveys, the average ages at
which boys and girls in the USA begin to smoke is 9.7 and 12.2 years respectively.
Cigarette use among high school seniors appears to have reached a peak in the
classes of 1976 and 1977, and is now on a downward trend, at least for men. In the
USA, the proportion of females who smoke now exceeds the proportion of males.
In most countries, the gender-specific differences in the distribution of smoking at
the age of adolescence or adulthood have levelled out over the past years.

The use of illegal drugs also begins during adolescence. In the USA, marijuana
use showed a dramatic rise during the 1960s and early 1970s. The data indicate
that since 1979 there has been no further increase. Obviously, marijuana use has
peaked for this age cohort. In contrast, there has been a slight upward trend in the
overall proportion of adolescents involved in other illicit drug use in the late 1970s.
From 1975 onward, just over one-fourth of males and females reported any use of
some illicit drug other than marijuana during the prior year. The most dramatic
shift in popularity involves cocaine (Bachman, Johnston, & O'Malley 1981, p.61).

In the FRG, as shown in the comparative study by Reuband (1988), 12% of all
14- to 17-year-old adolescents reported having experimented with illegal drugs in
1972 — in most cases, with marijuana. By 1982, this proportion had decreased to
5%. The proportions for the 18- to 20-year-olds were 12% and for the 21- to 24-
year-olds 16%. Most of the persons questioned reported having only tried
marijuana once or twice and therefore cannot be regarded as drug users. For many
of the young adults questioned, their experiences with drugs took place several
years earlier and are viewed as a passing phase in life. Compared with the USA,
we can speak of moderate experience with illegal drugs among adolescents.

Longitudinal comparisons show that in all Western countries the consumption
of illegal drugs has levelled out at a stable niveau, signalizing a phase of normaliza-
tion:

In the 1960s and 1970s illicit drug use emerged as an increasingly 'popular' form of deviance; so
instead of simply smoking cigarettes and using alcohol, many of today's teenagers also use
marijuana, and some use other illicit drugs. The emerging pattern of relationships with the use of
cocaine may illustrate our point particularly well. In 1975, cocaine use was low and was not very
strongly correlated with the background and lifestyle factors treated in this report. By 1979,
usage levels were higher and the correlations were much stronger; however, the patterns of correlation were the familiar ones consistently in evidence for alcohol, marijuana, and other illicit

drugs taken as a group. In other words, the kinds of young people most 'at risk' tend to remain much the same, while the kinds and amounts of substances used shift somewhat from year to year. (Bachman, Johnston, & O'Malley 1981, p.67)

The small decline in substance abuse is hardly grounds for complacency. Large numbers of adolescents still are involved with illegal drugs, and the percentages of those who abuse alcohol and/or cigarettes are indeed alarming. The data reported indicate that a large minority of high school seniors drink heavily on a daily basis. The data on adolescent tobacco use are still troubling. Deaths from lung cancer in women now exceed those from breast cancer and are accelerating at nearly double the rate of increase for men. The data indicate that at least one-quarter of high school seniors continue to smoke cigarettes on a daily basis (Johnston, O'Malley, & Bachman 1986; Bachman, Johnston, O'Malley, & Humphrey 1988).

A specific form of "drug consumption" is the use and abuse of medical and pharmaceutical substances. If a medicine is taken extremely often or in large quantities in the absence of medical indication, we can speak of drug abuse. In such cases, the medication is taken, for example, in order to strengthen or increase the organism's capacity for achievement or adaptation in respect to individual or social expectations. The medication is taken without supervision and is used in order to manipulate physical and psychological states. Thus, the patterns of consumption are comparable to those of other drugs.

The following groups of medicines/drugs are particularly open to abuse in all age groups:

1. Analgesics, that work by reducing the sensitivity to pain by interrupting neural connections. Chronic abuse leads to mental and, ocassionally, to physical dependence, and to liver and kidney diseases.
2. Stimulants, that essentially act by increasing the activity of the central nervous system and thus raise physical and psychological performance. Chronic abuse leads to mental dependence, sleeplessness, aggressivity, and heart diseases.
3. Tranquilizers, that work by inhibiting brain centers and thus induce a general reduction in activity and a readiness to sleep. Chronic abuse leads to psychological and, ocassionally, physical dependence, and reduces the ability to concentrate and to react.
4. Sedatives, that lessen the activity of the central nervous system. If taken in high doses, these substances increase the readiness to sleep and lead to psychological and physical dependence, permanent tiredness, depression, and delusions.

Many studies point to a noticeable increase in the distribution of medical and pharmaceutical substances within recent years. According to figures from the FRG, among the adult population the one-year prevalence rates of the consumption of substances are estimated as follows: analgesics, 41%; stimulants, 10%; tranquilizers, 22%; and sedatives, 19%. For the group of 15- to 17-year-old adolescents, the appropriate rates are 50% for analgesics, 9% for stimulants, and 11% for tranquilizers and sedatives (Engel & Hurrelmann 1988).

As recent research demonstrates, we have a development towards a "medicalization" of deviant and problem behavior (Conrad & Schneider 1980). Medicines are taken in order to suppress psychological problem behavior: During childhood and adolescence, parents and doctors overreact to social and psychological problem behavior (learning deficits, hyperactivity, aggressiveness, retardation) by resorting to the use of pharmacological substances. During adulthood, many persons make the attempt to suppress disorders and to impede the capacities for achievement and enjoyment by using medicines. Pharmaceutical drug abuse, therefore, is a specific form of symbolic expression of the psychological "costs" of the modern way of life under discussion here.

Chapter 3 Risk Factors: Stressors in the Life Course

In this chapter, I will systematically pursue the search for possible "risk factors," for the likely causes and conditions of different types of disorders. In its modern version, the term "risk factor" was developed in the area of stress research. In contrast to the concept of "cause" it takes into account the fact that it is not always possible to find one specific explanation for the appearance of the chronic disease typical of our time. Usually, no specific isolated source can be identified as the cause of illness, which could be treated with appropriate medication or surgery (Kaplan 1983).

Recent research agrees on the fact that not only physiological and physical features can act as risk factors, but also psychological disposition and conditions, as well as the social and ecological environment. Usually it is a specific combination, one could say the cumulative interaction of various risk factors, which acts as a starting point for pathological effects (Rabkin & Struening 1976; Kobasa 1979; Snyder & Ford 1987).

The term "risk factor" signifies the calculable risk that a person within a specific personal and/or environmental situation will get a specific disorder or disease within a specified period. If a statistically significant difference exists between this risk and the risk of a person who is not in this characteristic situation, then this characteristic situation or feature is called a risk factor. The introduction of this term into medical, psychological, and social epidemiology had an eminently practical significance: By using this term, preventive measures for eliminating or reducing risk factors became possible — independently of the state of the discussion on causal factors. Accordingly, elimination of the risk factor also means reducing the risk of becoming ill, at least in those cases where no irreversible damage has occurred (Pflanz 1973, p.13; Cassel 1975; Mausner & Kramer 1985).

In this chapter, following the modern stress paradigm, I will attempt to identify the most important kinds of stressors — as potential risk factors — for social, psychological, and physiological disorders in the three main life phases childhood, adolescence, and adulthood. In order to do this, I will use an exemplary form for the presentation. No attempt will be made to discuss exhaustively the voluminous individual studies on the various types of stressors and related symptoms. Instead, the most marked features for each life phase will be placed in the foreground of the discussion.

Stressors in Childhood

As far as potential risk factors are concerned, the living conditions of preschool children can be described in most industrialized countries as follows.

Today's families typically show a very broad spectrum of structural features. If one can speak of a single trend at all, then it is that the majority of families living in industrial societies are relatively small systems. They mostly consist only of father, mother, and one, or, two children. Furthermore, the number of single-parent families is on the upsurge, caused by the instability of marriage and the high divorce rate. Statistically, one out of three marriages will end in divorce in Western European countries; in North America, the rate is close to 40%.

In a growing minority of families, reliable social and psychological childcare, emotional contact with the child, and consideration for the needs and require-ments of the child can no longer be guaranteed, because of the organizational problems connected with instable partnerships and marriages. This tendency is reinforced through increasing numbers of mothers working outside of the home (Borman 1982; Laosa & Sigel 1982; Mattejat 1985; Sussman & Steinmetz 1987).

The modern family, as the institution mainly responsible for child rearing, is in a difficult position and depends increasingly on the creation of supportive public facilities such as kindergartens and daycare centers. The deeper reason for this lies in the high degree of individualization of lifestyles in industrial societies. The clas-sical model of the ideal middle-class (bourgeois) family, in which marriages lasted a lifetime, with the husband as the breadwinner of the family and its representa-tive in the outer world, and the wife responsible for the housework, child rearing, and for the interaction within the family, is now only applicable to a minority of about 40% of families.

The upcoming ideal of the new family of today is characterized by both parents working outside of the home on an equal basis, and each doing his or her fair share of the housework and child rearing; furthermore, each person is free to choose his or her own social contacts, which may even include extramarital relationships. In reality, women are clearly at a disadvantage in all areas when it comes to develop-ing to their full potential. The marriage is in danger when the ideal of fair partner-ship is disregarded for longer periods of time. In most cases, it is the lack of com-mitment on the part of the men to this "new" construction that endangers the mar-riage. If the parents separate, custody of the children is given to one of them, usu-ally the mother.

Separation of the Parents as Risk Factor

The great majority of children whose parents are divorced or separated are under great psychological and social stress, since it is difficult for the children to under-stand the factors which caused the relationship to fail, and that, furthermore, the children cannot grasp the full scope of the consequences which this rupture of the family will have on their lives (Rickel & La Rue 1987, p.59). The situation is usually complicated by the fact that the children are seldom properly informed about the impending changes and developments — thus, they are not able to develop preliminary coping strategies. On the contrary, children are often used as go-betweens, to bring contradictory or double-binding messages from one parent to the other. In this way, the children themselves may be involved in a situation marked by distorted communication and may, involuntarily, contribute to further complications in the relationship.

When parents separate, the child's contact with the parent with whom he/she lives remains intense, or becomes even more intense, whereas the relationship with the parent no longer living at home often breaks off completely. This, in turn, leads to intense feelings of loss, which are hard for the child to cope with, because the absent parent continues to exist socially and psychologically, but is unreachable for the child. Separation and divorce are profoundly stressful life-events which are associated with a wide range of physical and psychiatric symptomatology among affected adults and children. Survey data have consistently indicated greater happiness of married persons, compared with divorced or separated persons (Pearlin & Johnson 1977). It is easy to think of examples of exceptional mothers who maintained warm, cohesive homes while supporting their children, but it is not clear that these are representative of ordinary people who may be worn down by the heavy, continuous demands of work and child rearing, leading to the state of exhaustion and demoralization that is the precursor of physical and psychiatric illness (Dohrenwend et al. 1980).

The situation is further complicated by the heavy social and psychological pressure placed on the parent who has custody. As a rule, financial problems also arise, since it is more costly to run two households than one. In the FRG, for example, in 80% of the cases the children live with their mothers, and since the majority of mothers have no job outside the home, the financial situation deteriorates. The mother may be forced to look for a job, which means that the child is now also separated for longer periods of time from the remaining parent. The separation may also involve moving to a new neighborhood, in which case contacts with old friends and neighbors are lost. "Orphans of divorce" often feel psychologically stigmatized, and may react irritably, showing signs of behavioral disorders. If the parent who has custody gets involved with a new partner, complicated emotional conflicts may ensue in the relationship, especially if the new partner brings his or her own children into the family (Napp-Peters 1985).

Studies from the USA clearly confirm these trends. Separation from the absent parent takes its toll emotionally and financially on all members of the family, and young people can be hit especially hard. Measuring well-being in economic terms, statistics show that poverty is a growing reality in single-parent families. The number of persons below the poverty line living in families headed by a woman with no husband present jumped by 27% between 1979 and 1986. In 1985, 67% of single mothers with school-age children were in the labor force at least part-time or part-year. A single parent working at the minimum wage would have to support herself and two children at 20% below the official poverty line (Grant Commission 1987, p.14).

Material and Nonmaterial Deprivation as Risk Factors

Besides insecurity caused by separation and parents' involvement with their work — factors which exist for all professional groups — one must also focus on the risks to children's development posed by unfavorable material conditions, conditions which are also widespread in industrialized welfare states. Families can be pushed towards the borderline of financial subsistence and poverty through unemployment, long-term illness, crime, etc. Often, the results are tensions in the family, a broken home, aggressive and violent fights between family members, and uncontrolled disciplinary measures, which do not provide the necessary conditions for the children's social, psychological, and physical development.

Given the fact that in "normal" families the needs of the children are often viewed as tiresome because of the difficulty in reconciling child-raising on the one hand and work, housework, and leisure, on the other, it is easy to understand why in such extreme circumstances as those mentioned above, it often comes to a complete breakdown, in which the most elementary needs of the children are no longer taken care of; often the children are neglected or abused (Garbarino, Schellenbach, & Sebes 1986).

In their first years of life, children need reliable, stable, and predictable social structures in their relationships, which support and stimulate their personal development. Researchers studying families have drawn up the following list of criteria of favorable conditions in a child's first years of life (Schneewind, Beckmann, & Engfer 1983):

1. Stimulation, that is, confronting the child with objects and persons with which it must learn to cope
2. Appropriateness, that is, adjusting the level and the duration of the stimulation to the child's specific developmental phase
3. Variety, that is, providing the child with different kinds and qualities of stimulation through language, gestures, movement, and toys
4. Acceptance, that is, being willing to tolerate the individuality of the child, as it is concretely expressed in its behavior — within certain limits, of course, which must be respected
5. Responsiveness, that is, the consistent and appropriately differentiated feedback on the child's behavior
6. Affection, that is, the social, gestural, and physical demonstration of affection and care

In order to develop a positive feeling about themselves, to learn self-control, prosocial orientation, friendly and cooperative behavior with their peer group and adults, responsibility for themselves, and to develop their intellectual abilities, children need continuing support and warmth, consistent supervision by adults with a sensitive, explanatory approach to child rearing who, at the same time, are willing to let the child expand its horizon stepwise. This behavior can only manifest itself when the parents or other persons raising the child themselves live in satisfactory relationships, including favorable material conditions (Boyce 1985).

The quality of the relationship between the parents is an important factor. The relationship provides a good atmosphere in which the child's needs can be fulfilled — provided that it is emotionally positive, there is a balance of power in the relationship, and conflicts are solved. Furthermore, the interaction of the entire family as a unit is also important. Crucial features are the family's solidarity and adaptability to the stresses and challenges involved in different phases of the life cycle. Flexibility concerning rules, and the ability to do things together as a family are important features of a familial setting which gives each member his or her personal independence, encourages each member to be responsible for himself or herself, and, at the same time, is conducive to such goals. If these conditions are given, then the situation is favorable for coping flexibly and effectively with the challenges coming form the outside world (Pearlin & Johnson 1977; Laosa & Sigel 1982; Borman 1982; Cochran 1987).

In order to develop a healthy personality, children have specific requirements in their relationships, requirements which a large number of families cannot provide today, at least to a sufficient extent. Unhappy or conflict-ridden relationships in the family are a strong risk factor in the child's development. Financial problems, problems related to the mother's or father's job, an alcoholic parent, fighting between the parents, and other similar factors may directly impair a child's acquisition of behavioral competence. Different studies have shown that when tensions exist in the family, the quality of care given to the child by the mother or father and the emotional acceptance of the child is less than in control families (Garmezy & Rutter 1983; McCubbins, Sussman, & Patterson 1984; Garbarino, Schellenbach, & Sebes 1986). In families with unfavorable social status, stress situations lead more quickly to stressful constellations within the family. The stress is felt especially deeply when difficult constellations at school or in the neighborhood are added to those already existing in the family — often these affect each other mutually.

Over- and Understimulation as Risk Factors

The physical, psychological, and social developmental possibilities of children depend not only on the familial conditions discussed above, but also on the social and ecological living conditions outside of the family. An area where these two domains overlap is housing, which has a strong influence on the spatial organization of family life. Even in those places where housing provides adequate space, it is rarely adapted to meet the sensory and motor needs of small children; instead, as far as functionality and esthetic standards are concerned, it is usually oriented towards the requirements of adults.

Because of their physical and spatial environment, today's children are highly dependent on the training of their optical and acoustic perception; radios, television, videos, walkmen, etc. lead to overstimulation of these senses, whereas their emotional and psychomotoric capacities are, in part, not sufficiently stimulated; they are virtually handicapped as far as certain emotional and physical experiences are concerned. The children's ability to acquire sensual experience is often strongly regulated and channeled through neighborhoods with no green, open spaces, through artificial building materials, equipment, and toys, and through lack of body contact invested with emotion. In contrast to this, the audiovisual and print media often present sensational and intensely stimulating experiences which, seen qualitatively and quantitatively, do not always contribute to a realistic assessment of social reality (Borman 1982).

The following areas of experience and activities can be identified as causing recognizeable damage to children's physical, psychological, and social development:

1. Traffic: It has expanded so greatly and has become so complex that children can no longer assess it appropriately. The major cause of child and juvenile deaths is traffic accidents; damage caused by accidents has reached shocking proportions (Hawton 1986).
2. Lack of space for physical expression: In the kindergartens and at home in the family, inappropriate spatial facilities hinder one of the basic functions of child development, a hindrance which can deeply disturb the spiritual and psychological development of the young. Consequences of this may be impairment of physical capacities and motor development, as well as psychological disorders.
3. Environmental stress: Here, only a few conditions specific to children can be identified; however, pollution of the air, water, and soil, and high noise levels are certainly no less of a health hazard for children than for adolescents and adults.
4. Nutrition: In this area the emphasis is on the issue of being underweight or overweight, and on physiologically harmful nutrition. A special problem here is the tendency toward the consumption of foods rich in calories and high in sugar content.
5. Rhythm of daily life: Because of frequent changes in persons caring for the small child, and being kept in different institutions, most small children typically experience their daily life as fragmented, partly accompanied by irritable reactions. The family's daily time-schedule is oriented upon outside factors like the parent's work hours or the daycare center's opening hours, and other factors which stucture time and living space, creating excessive regulation. Furthermore, the daily routines and activities in the kindergartens and daycare centers are often problematic, too: many of these children are often forced to perform an entire agenda of work, learning, and play programs, which brings more stress, regulation, and nervousness than the learning-by-doing experiences actually intended with this agenda.

The effects of all of these risk factors from outside of the family may remain latent for many years; their consequences only become apparent much later in life. This is why it is so difficult to shed light on the cause-effect relationship. Often, problem-causing living conditions will not be taken seriously until the children show massive reactions like psychological and/or physiological disorders.

Acutely Stressful Life-Events as Risk Factors

Since the 1960s, work studying stressful events has become an important research domain of social psychiatry and clinical psychology, as well as of sociology. Critical events are classified as "stressors," that is, as stress factors which require a considerable amount of adjustment from the person in question. The necessary adjustment cannot be made if specific events occur at the same time and with great intensity. As a reaction to this the probability for social, psychological, or physical disorders increases (Dohrenwend & Dohrenwend 1974).

Checklists of experiences which can create critical situations for children (taken from research results on adults) have been drawn up (Johnson 1986). A seven-point scale is used, with the last point 7 standing for "most alarming" and 1 standing for "least alarming." For grade-school children the following factors have been identified, listed according to the amount of stress identified with the factor:

1. Death of a parent
2. Having to repeat a school year
3. Physical violence between the parents
4. Being caught stealing
5. Being suspected of lying
6. Having disciplinary action taken by the teacher
7. Having an operation
8. Getting lost
9. Getting laughed at by the class
10. Moving to another school
11. Having a nightmare
12. Not being able to do all of one's homework
13. Being the last one chosen for a team
14. Being on the losing team in a competition

Since many studies have shown that besides the perceptions of the individuals involved, the social environment in which life-altering experiences occur also plays a very important role, many researchers have developed lists in which the individual's subjective assessment is included; furthermore, the individual is asked to evaluate the effects of the experiences which altered his of her life (Johnson 1986, p.40).

Researchers were able to establish a relationship between a broad spectrum of psychological disorders and physical impairments in stressful living situations. Various studies were able to establish a relationship between the number of stressful experiences and psychophysiological disorders. It seems that the children's physiological immunological system is also affected by their living conditions. The body is more likely to develop antibodies in less stressful living conditions than in acute states of crisis. This has been proven for illnesses like influenza, tonsilitis, pneumonia, and bronchitis. Severe stress like the death of a parent or accidents reduce the body's defence mechanism, also in the physiological domain (Henry 1982; Butler & Corner 1984; Rickel & Allen 1987, p.67).

We do not yet know very much about the interacting mechanisms between psychological stress and physical illness. Researchers suspect that under the influence of different stressors, the brain sends specific types of hormones (neuropeptides) into the blood stream, from where they influence the central nervous system, as well as the heart, stomach, and digestive functions; furthermore, they ensure that greater or lesser resistance to disturbance and illnesses occurs. These "stress hormones" are efficient messengers between the brain and the different organs.

As shown by the research mentioned in this area, the relationship between stressful experiences and physical disorders is not mechanical. Therefore, in order to understand this interaction, it is only partially effective to add up critical experiences, isolated from the other factors. On the contrary, the individual's subjective assessment of the stress situation and his/her ability to cope is decisive. This ability depends on different personal dispositions — both physical and psychological, including locus of control, language skills, physical constitution, temperament, different styles of perception, as well as retarded or accelerated physical and psychological development (Farran & Cooper 1986).

The existence of risk factors does not allow us to establish simple cause and effect relationships. Some factors only produce an effect in conjunction with specific other factors, and their effect can be changed to a great degree by personal and social moderator variables. A person's social environment can either intensify the risk factors or counterbalance them. On the whole, the importance of the effects of risk factors can only be established in a longitudinal analysis.

It is important to consider the interaction between biological and psychosocial stressors in future research. For example, such an analysis could explain why young boys are much more susceptible to stress than young girls. Instead of only focusing on genetic or environmental factors, it would be much more productive for scientific research to include the category of "temperament" in these considerations — a category which combines elements from both groups of factors (Chess & Thomas 1986).

Apparently, the following features can all be used to differentiate between boys and girls: irritability, excitability, regularity of biological rhythms, ability to be distracted, emotionality, and readiness to make contacts with others. Most studies concur in the view that boys are more dependent than girls on variables concerning temperament. It seems as if male infants are more susceptible to pre- and postnatal disturbances than are female infants. Although boys are permitted to be more aggressive than girls, it seems, at the same time, as if the views on what is considered normal "male" behavior are quite rigid. In any case, it appears that maladjustment reactions to social norms, a disturbed relationship to sexual identity and emotional and cognitive disturbance are more common with boys than with girls in early childhood. The same applies to aggressiveness and hyperactivity (Kessler & McLeod 1984; Condry 1984; Rossi 1985; Petersen & Ebata 1987).

Thus, in order to explain the development of social, physical, and psychological disorders we have to take into consideration the child's personal characteristics as well as the conditions of the social environment as specific intervening variables. Usually, the personal features are of great importance, but it also becomes clear that a child's specific susceptibilities or resilience only come into play when specific other, additional environmental factors appear. The personality variables determine how great is the need for stability from the environment, for stimulation, for emotional acceptance, etc. It is only through the interaction of these factors that the further development of a child can be explained (Werner & Smith 1982; Roberts & Peterson 1984).

Stressors in Adolescence

Historical studies show that "adolescence" only came to be considered as a specific, independent phase in the human life cycle during the second half of the last century. The creation of adolescence is closely related to the economic, political, and cultural changes which took place during industrialization — one of these changes being the establishment of a compulsory school system. In the last hundred years (only 3 or 4 generations), the criteria for achieving the social status of adulthood have changed fundamentally. It is above all in the three important areas listed below that the structural features of the status passage have changed considerably:

1. In the schools and job training
2. In the social relationships with the family of origin
3. In leisure time, including social contacts with the peer group

Status Insecurity as a Risk Factor

In all industrialized nations, one can observe a continuing process in which the phases spent in school and on job training are growing longer in the individual's biography. The time at which young people enter the job market is being extended. Attending a school and then, afterwards, a college or university in order to get job training (which often extends into the individual's third decade) has become the dominant feature of adolescence. On the one hand, the younger generation's chances of obtaining a high level of education and job training have risen enormously through this process of "educational expansion." On the other hand, however, the competition for obtaining a favorable starting position for the transition into professional life has become much more fierce. In order to have the same social status as the family of origin, many adolescents today must obtain diplomas which, in many cases, are much more advanced than those obtained by their parents. At the same time, having a high-level diploma (from school, job training, or the university) is by no means a guarantee today for obtaining a high-level job with favorable chances for promotion (Hurrelmann 1987b).

The everyday living conditions of adolescents are touched by these changes in the structural features. Even in Western Europe, where this is a quite new phenomenon, having a job is no longer a characteristic feature of adolescence for those under 20. The transition into professional life — that is, into a very important feature of adulthood — has been prolonged into the twenties for the great majority of young people. Work, which in Europe was a typical feature of adolescence at the beginning of this century, has been replaced by school or vocational training. At the same time, the transitional process into the job market is becoming increasingly difficult to plan and calculate (Hurrelmann & Engel 1989).

The experience of being a useful member of society through one's work, of learning about the norms of economic, rational efficiency in factories and offices, and of learning to provide for oneself financially can now only be made relatively late in life, because young people enter the job market so much later. Although school provides them with intellectual and social stimulation, it is an area in which few experiences with responsibility for oneself and for other persons are possible; furthermore, solidarity cannot often be experienced there; the student is under strong pressure to succeed individually, and typically, abstract learning processes are predominant in schools (Hurrelmann 1984a, b).

European authors have maintained that this restructuring of adolescents' experiences from a lifestyle primarily integrated into work, or at least oriented to work, to one primarily determined by the school cannot remain without consequences on the developmental processes of adolescents and their attitudes towards society and employment. Because they enter professional life so much later than previous generations, today's adolescents have great individual freedom in how they spend their time, in their choice of partners and means of communication, and in how they arrange their daily lives, especially as far as the mass media and consumer industry are concerned. For technical and economic reasons, all development in industrial societies tends toward eliminating the process of socialization of adolescents in and through work, and instead replaces this process with learning activities which become more and more abstract. It seems that this process is irreversible, for it is precisely in the newer production technologies that technical know-how and the mechanisms by which they function can no longer be learned in the concrete situation, on the job (Baethge 1989).

Long periods of time spent in school or on job training have become a requirement, but not necessarily a guarantee — that is, ensuring status — for the classical, main role of adulthood: having a job and supporting oneself. Due to the insecurities involved in adolescents' transitions from school into the labor force, the possibility of experiencing work and one's profession as a suitable basis for the creation of identity and, consequently, developing appropriate perspectives for one's life and work is being questioned. The repercussions which the ongoing crisis in the job market have on the educational system as an important agent of socialization have led to a continuing separation of job training from job perspectives and, thus, to a crisis concerning the importance of schooling.

Unstable Social Integration as a Risk Factor

The features which we have described have clearly affected the psychological and social relationship which adolescents have with their family of origin: On the one hand, adolescents leave the parental home at a much later date than did the generation before them, because longer phases of job training mean longer economic dependence on the parents. On the other hand, today's adolescents develop at an early age a way of living (as far as leisure and consumption is concerned) which is independent from that of their parents; they move into their own apartments or share living quarters with others from their peer group, and they also move in with partners of the opposite sex at an earlier age.

The process of separating from the parents takes place in different dimensions and at different times, thus sometimes creating complex situations in the family of origin. This is also intensified by the fact that the family only consists of a few persons, who are connected to each other by a close network of emotions. Accordingly, the importance of the family as an economic supplier and a backbone for social support is very pronounced for adolescents today, whereas its importance for determining living arrangements, lifestyle, and partnerships has decreased significantly (Youniss 1980).

It is typical of all industrial societies that the peer group takes over the function of socialization at a relatively early stage in the individual's personal development. Peer groups (whose members meet in their free time) are characterized by the fact that they give their members valuable possibilities for participation, possibilities which the remaining domains — especially school and the family — cannot provide in such a scope. This is the reason why they are so important for the psychological and social orientation of young adolescents (Youniss 1980).

The importance of the peer group presumably grows in proportion to the degree of social separation between adolescent and parents. In this difficult phase of separation, the peer group can take over the function of acting as a psychological support for the adolescent until a new type of relationship between the adolescent and his or her parents can be established. Furthermore, the peer group plays an important role in determining how the adolescent organizes his/her leisure time and his/her activities as a consumer. The peer group sets the standards upon which adolescents orient their consumer activities; thus, it provides an effective code of behavior for adolescents. Peer groups often create a youth culture, which permits the development of an independent lifestyle separate from that of the adults. In this sense, peer groups act as an important medium for permitting adolescents to demonstrate independence (Biddle, Bank, & Marlin 1980).

In the areas of friendship, consumption, media, and intimate relationships with a partner, adolescents typically have a great deal of freedom in their lives. This constellation gives them freedom for their individual development and for discovering themselves and their own goals; furthermore, it permits them a high degree of autonomy, spontaneity, creativity, and individuality. This freedom is used imaginatively by many adolescents to explore possibilities for making decisions and finding alternatives and for creating an individual lifestyle. Their taste in fashion and clothes, music and leisure activities, language, and political expression is proof of an independent way of life, in part independent from adults. Adolescents are able to develop forms of adapting and coping with social reality which provide them with a broad range of sensual, esthetic, emotional, interactive, and communicative experiences (Murphy & Moriarty 1976).

The financial resources which today's adolescents have are, on the average, often quite comfortable in comparison with the generation of their parents. With the exception of fringe groups, adolescents are financially well-off and fulfill a multitude of wishes in the areas of leisure time and consumption, which were unobtainable for their parents. However, this seemingly high degree of freedom in the area of leisure and consumption is illusionary, for this sector — which is strongly determined by commercial interests — only permits limited meaningful development of the adolescent's personality. A further problem may also be hidden behind the adolescent's comfortable financial situation: money is an unstable element in life, even for adolescents, because it is used to make comparisons and to awaken competition in the peer group. Being financially well-to-do is conducive to envious comparisons among adolescents and, thus, it is a serious source of psychological and social stress, which can lead to considerable irritation in this malleable phase of youthful personality development (Engel & Hurrelmann 1988).

Thus, adolescents are placed into a difficult situation between the (seemingly) "free" leisure area and the "regulated" area of schooling and job training. They "buy" their freedom by spending a lot of time in highly regulated educational programs, in which normed expectations of achievement are directed at them. Adolescents develop their individuality in a tense living situation in an affluent society, which at any time can signal to them that its multitude of colorful products cannot be counted on.

Today, adolescents have a wide range of possibilities for expanding their individuality. But neither parents nor teachers can promise them that chances and opportunities for a future with interesting perspectives and for personal identity will grow out of these possibilities, for the social horizon of the future is very difficult to plan and to calculate for adolescents. There are no guaranteed pespectives for the future or calculable possibilities for job or life planning. No one can promise adolescents a fair future — the prolongation of education can lead to permanent unemployment; good educational possibilities are often offered within the framework of educational programs which are, objectively speaking, devoid of perspectives for the future (Hurrelmann 1984a); the great amount of time devoted to finding oneself and to introspection can lead to tortured speculation on the meaning of life. At a time in their lives when they are still forming their personality, adolescents are confronted with a multitude of possibilities, but also with many frustrations and a great deal of insecurity.

Risk Constellations for Delinquency

There are many indications which point to the fact that the living situation of adolescents described here can be the origin of the development of physical, psychological, and social symptoms of disorders in adolescence. In a representative study of adolescents in the FRG, Engel and Hurrelmann (1988) discovered the following trends concerning social deviance:

1. Social deviance can be found above all in the group of adolescents who are in a difficult position as far as school performance and high educational expectations on the part of the parents are concerned. If pressure caused by parental expectations concerning their child's school performance is very high and if it becomes apparent that parental expectations cannot be met, many adolescents seem to react with deviant behavior. Adolescents who list conflict with their parents in different areas are also those with a higher probability of developing delinquency. Delinquency thus is a by-product of conflict with the parents and indicates that the separation from the parental home is difficult and not yet completed.
2. Deviance is connected with difficult integration processes into the peer group. If adolescents do not succed at being accepted by their peer group as they wish to be, and to assume an undisputed social position as members of the group, and if they suffer from lack of popularity and insufficient recognition from their peer group, this may result in considerable insecurity in their social orientation and self-estimation. Problem behavior like aggression, stealing, and vandalism can be seen as an "instrument" with which the adolescent attempts to demonstrate that he or she belongs to the peer group. Here we can clearly see how certain forms of problem behavior are intensely related to elementary processes of social integration (Jessor & Jessor 1977).

These research findings are corroborated by different studies which prove that criminal behavior is the final link in a long chain of stress, caused by unfavorable socialization in the family, lack of success at school, no school-leaving certificate, none or insufficient professional training, and unemployment. According to the latest research, criminal behavior must be seen as a reaction to such deprivation. The high and still growing proportion of adolescents involved in the total crime statistics must be taken seriously as an indication of increasing social and psychological marginalization of a minority of adolescents, and must be viewed above all as a reaction to underprivileged living conditions and unfavorable conditions of socialization, as well as being proof of barriers and ruptures in the process of social integration. Adolescents who resort to this kind of behavior obviously cannot find any other way to deal with the demands placed on them in different areas of social activity. At school, they cannot achieve socially recognized results, thus, they find no confirmation of themselves at school, and there is no corresponding development of a socially acceptable lifestyle in other areas. Typically, these adolescents turn to the peer group as a resort in which a feeling of belonging and being accepted can be experienced (Siegel & Senna 1981).

Risk Constellations for Psychological Disorders

As has been said, adolescence can be described as a transitional phase in life, characterized by intense and accelerated changes in the demands placed upon the young person. Development in such a transitional phase in considered as being appropriate and successful if the adolescent is confronted with well-dosed changes and situational demands. If this is the case, the transitional phase can be used effectively to "reprogram" and to extend the existing behavioral repertoire. Successfully meeting demands creates a new constellation, which the adolescent himself/herself perceives as stimulating. Demands are seen as challenges which are met in a productive way (Havighurst 1956).

If, however, demands are placed upon the adolescent which transcend his or her current behavioral repertoire and which put too great a burden on the coordination of the various behavioral programs in the different developmental areas, then there is the danger that the situation will be dealt with unsuccessfully which, in turn, may lead to the appearance of repressive tendencies, avoidance, and behavioral disorders (Coleman 1980).

Accordingly, disturbances and serious crises in personality development occur above all when changes in different areas of development do not take place in a forseeable sequence, but all at once, at a specific moment in development. The multitude of developmental tasks in adolescence requires active efforts towards adjustment and active efforts for coping in different areas, in order to construct behavioral programs for coping with the current demands.

The very nature of adolescence as a transitional phase requires that the adolescent relinquish old perspectives on his/her environment and himself/herself in the different areas of development and acquire totally new ones. At the same time, a reorientation of behavioral patterns and the attitudes and effects which accompany these patterns must take place. If the scope of the demands reaches a level which surmounts the individual's potential for coping, then serious crisis and disorders may occur. The social, cognitive, emotional, and normative programs for coping with the new situation cannot meet the demands placed upon them and are overloaded, as far as their potential is concerned (Coleman 1980).

Thus, it can happen frequently in adolescence (as we have shown above) that, through disturbances in concentration and performance, different types of deficits converge over a longer period of time, causing an ongoing overburdening of the individual's capacities for coping (Cullinan, Epstein, & Lloyd 1983, p.255):

1. Inability to concentrate on cognitive tasks and to learn step by step
2. Inability to establish and maintain satisfying social relationships with teachers
3. Inability in socially normal teaching situations to demonstrate what is considered to be appropriate behavior
4. Inability to establish an appropriate self-image, to define social situations flexibly, and to tolerate frustration
5. Inability to accept performance deficits with emotionally stable reactions without succumbing to depression

In adolescence, problems with school performance and difficulty with concentration are closely related to social or psychological disturbance of normal personality development. These disturbances can be the real cause of problems at school; they may also be a reaction to problems with school performance. Whereas problems with concentration and with school performance are observed more often in adolescents from families with higher socioeconomic status, other symptoms of psychological disorders as identified by psychiatrists occur more frequently in the lower status families: among them problems in making contact, problems in adjustment, and overactivity. As one can see in Petri's (1979) results, listed in Table 4, children from the upper and/or the middle classes are — in comparison — more frequently listed in the registration forms of psychiatric clinics with the following symptoms: overadjustment, failure at school, depression, and psychosomatic disorders.

It seems as if adolescents from families with low social status tend more towards aggressive and conflict-oriented forms of behavior. These behavioral patterns suggest that these adolescents perceive themselves as underprivileged in comparison with others where their chances for development are concerned. In contrast to this, symptoms of interiorization abound in the upper and middle classes. On the whole, there are quantitatively more disorders in the lower social classes, which would indicate an interrelation between unfavorable educational opportunities, a bad economic situation, and scare possibilities for leisure time activities (Kessler & Cleary 1980).

These results are supported by the classic studies of Hollingshead and Redlich (1958) as well as Srole, Langner, Michael, Opler, and Rennie (1962). These studies document the inverse relationship between social class and most forms of psychological disorder and mental illness.

Table 4. Class background and psychological disorders (1040 patients between the ages of 6–18 from the division of child and adolescent psychiatry of the University Hospital, Berlin), figures in percent (Petri 1979)

Total	Lower classes (n = 354)	Middle classes (n = 528)	Upper classes (n = 158)
Problems establishing contact	54.0	45.1	44.9
Conduct disorders	34.7	26.1	25.3
Overactivity	28.2	21.4	22.2
Fearfulness	26.6	25.2	17.1
Taking things/stealing	16.9	10.2	11.4
Heightened aggressiveness	16.1	11.6	7.6
Overadjustment	12.7	17.4	10.1
Failure at school	29.9	27.5	38.0
Depression	12.1	17.2	20.2
Moodiness	10.2	12.5	17.1
Digestive problems	6.5	8.3	13.3
Stomach problems	6.2	6.4	11.4

It is obviously the case that children and adolescents who come from families which are financially and socially deprived have a harder time coping with stress than children and adolescents who grow up in better conditions. Socially under-privileged families are less effective in developing forms and strategies for coping with stress. Observations have shown that families which are more privileged socially, and which have generally more positive experiences in coping with difficult situations, have greater resistance towards factors which endanger the mental health of its members. People from socially privileged families have more financial resources and more power and influence, by means of which they are better able to cope with stress situations (Wirsching & Stierlin 1982).

Most studies of this type place the emphasis on the vertical ranking of individuals on each indicator of social class. In the studies of this tradition, a model of social class is applied: Individuals are ranked according to their relationship to patterns of production, consumption, and power. Status is defined as a dimension of prestige or social honor possessed by individuals or groups; it is an evaluation of their social esteem.

The fact that adolescents usually occupy contradictory positions on different indicators of status at the same time may, however, be of additional importance for the transitory character of the phase of life called adolescence. Recent research has shown that the person occupying different ranks of different status indicators (education, financial resources, prestige, etc.) may have conflicting expectations about others' demands and uncertainty about his or her own behavior. Dressler (1988), in a study of emotional distress, could show significant interrelations between a "lifestyle incongruity" of this type and the manifestation of a psychiatric symptomatology in a black population. Because barriers to upward social mobility have been relaxed gradually for Afro-Americans only over the past 30 years, there are significant numbers of persons for whom education, occupation, and style of life are not linked closely. Discrepancies among these dimensions predict psychological disorders. In the black community, because of the unequal distribution of wealth, people have less access to those occupations necessary for upward mobility and hence for congruity with the culturally valued lifestyle. At the same time, however, the overall ideology of American culture, shared by many members of the black community, is one of open access to avenues of upward mobility. This study points to several problems that may be typical for the adolescent phase of life in general (Hurrelmann, Engel, Holler, & Nordlohne 1988).

Risk Constellations for Suicide

Studies on suicide list three main sources of stress found in connection with suicide and attempted suicide in adolescence:

1. Tense or severed social relationships with the parents, often caused by conflicts, separation, or divorce of the parents
2. Poor academic performance at school impending failure at school, or the experience of having failed at school

3. Crises in relationships with peers, especially social isolation in the peer group, and problems in establishing relationships with the opposite sex (Diekstra & Hawton 1987)

Accordingly, the tendency to commit suicide, or the actual suicide itself, are the result of each individual's personal forms of coping with the demands which life makes, with developmental tasks and psychological and social stress situations. Suicide is usually the end of a long chain of events which have led to serious structural disturbances of a person's belief in himself/herself and his or her worth as a human being, and a crisis in personal development. Symptoms accompanying a suicidal intent are: prolonged sadness, behavioral problems, disturbed sleeping and/or eating patterns, poor academic performance, death of a loved one, family problems, expressed feelings of worthlessness or hopelessness, the presence of depressive illness as opposed to the normal ups and downs of adolescence, social alienation of the adolescent, and overwhelming and intolerable anxiety, which can build up over a matter of days or even hours prior to a suicide attempt (Berman 1986).

The following factors play a key role in the attempt to explain how suicides occur: the degree of personal stability, self-confidence, and a sense of continuity in oneself vis-à-vis different situations in life and different phases of life. A positive self-image is a necessity for healthy personality development. A negative self-image is, as a rule, a sign of psychological insecurity and instability. Each individual must go through a difficult process in which identity and self-worth are coordinated. This coordination can be considered as established when conflicts with the individual's inner and outer world have led to viable solutions (Erikson 1959; Murphy & Moriarty 1976).

Adolescence is a developmental phase in life when, for the first time, these demands on the adolescent's personality are intensified; demands which, under our present conditions, drive an increasing number of adolescents to desperation. The predominant opportunity structures in several countries objectively render difficult the establishment and maintenance of a positive self-image: Adolescents experience the tension between the freedom found in the areas of consumption and leisure and the restrictions found in school or job-training programs and occupational chances. The more sensitive and vulnerable adolescents suffer from a lack of positive options for the future and/or often experience — occasionally very directly and very personally in their own body and mind — the threats to peace and the environment.

If these highly sensitive adolescents are plunged into stress situations or crises through disturbance of their social relationships or critical life-events, they can fall into deep depressions and become so thoroughly demoralized that they resort to suicide. A characteristic feature of suicide is an unfavorable constellation in which the adolescent's personal and psychological resources are depleted at the same time as social resources are exhausted: a flexible, active style of coping with problems is missing, while, at the same time, there is no reliable, continuing support from the social network of relationships (Peck, Faberow, & Litman 1985).

Risk Constellations for Drug Addiction

As many studies show, alcohol consumption in adolescence is promoted through unfavorable socialization conditions in the family, especially if the parents raise their children with a great deal of surveillance and restrictions, and through an unfavorable emotional climate in the family. Adolescents who have not learned to deal with conflicts productively, but instead have learned to deny their existence or repress them, are more in danger of becoming addicted to alcohol than are adolescents who are able to actively come to terms with their daily problems (Jessor & Jessor 1977; Bachman, O'Malley & Johnston 1982).

Pertinent studies have proven the existence of psychological mechanisms like denial and repression in the area of school performance, that is, in a central social area of experience. Conflicts at school, which, as a rule, are related to school performance, become a serious problem for those adolescents who, already as children, only learned few or insufficient or inapplicable strategies for coping with school. Alcohol, as a false means of "dealing" with situations (a means which is easily accessible in our culture) is used more quickly and more intensely by pupils with undifferentiated forms of behavior than by other pupils. As a rule, these pupils are not aware of their own motivation for drinking akohol, that is, as a means for dealing with conflicts and of compensating for failure (Engel, Nordlohne, Hurrelmann, & Holler 1988).

These findings are confirmed by the fact that adolescents who have marked problems with their self-esteem are more frequently in danger of becoming addicted to alcohol. The more negatively students see their school performance, the greater their fear of school, and therefore, the greater their tendency to consume alcohol in order to deal with their fear. In contrast to this, there is little tendency to manipulate one's mood with alcohol and other drugs when school performance is positive. Fear and rejection of school must thus be seen as a form of individual tension, toward which the adolescent reacts with the drug alcohol.

Additionally, one must keep in mind the social pressure associated with alcohol in our society. In the studies mentioned above, the majority of adolescents indicated that they were put under considerable social pressure in their circles of friends if they refused alcohol. Alcohol is seen as a means of improving bad moods, overcoming difficulties in having contact with others, and reducing social or sexual inhibitions. Male adolescents often perceive alcohol as a type of game for testing strength; it is seen as a ritual enactment of togetherness in the peer group. Particularly excessive consumption of alcohol can thus be the result of group pressure (Kandel 1980; Kandel, Kessler, & Margulies 1978; Silbereisen, Eyferth, & Rudinger 1986).

Obviously, consumption of tobacco is also closely linked to personality and fulfills various subjective needs as well as instrumental, social, and symbolic functions in the developmental process. An important factor in adolescent smoking is having prestige in the peer group or circle of friends: Group members smoke demonstratively in order to attain more prestige and to compensate for low social status. Vice versa, students who smoke can act as models and, because they are viewed as being powerful, lead other group members into smoking.

A longitudinal study by Wills (1985) shows significant connections between the degree of social integration in the peer group and the degree to which the peer group is used for social relations and entertainment on the one hand, and tobacco consumption on the other. At the same time, a negative correlation was established between the degree of perceived social support through parents and other adults and tobacco consumption. These findings prove that tobacco consumption and the ability to establish social relationships are closely linked. Furthermore, the nature of tobacco consumption as a social act is also expressed by the fact that most adolescents smoke their first cigarette in the company of a friend. The percentage of smokers is especially high when the adolescent's friends also smoke; the same applies to parents, brothers, and sisters.

Tobacco consumption is a form of behavior which is specific to certain social classes. Adolescents from families with low socioeconomic status have a noticeably higher rate of consumption. In these social groups, smoking is perceived as an expression of belonging to the group and as a form of behavior which shows adjustment and integration into the norms and values of the group. Consumption of the legal drug tobacco is thus related to patterns of daily living, becoming itself a part of daily life (Johnston, O'Malley, & Bachman 1986).

The same applies to the use of illegal drugs: It is woven into the fabric of the adolescent's biography, and involves the entire structure of his or her life. According to current studies, the tendency towards drug consumption increases when the range of experiences decreases and the adolescent has deficits in his or her world of experiences. Adolescents who have too few activities in daily life which in themselves bring satisfaction will attempt to improve their self-esteem in order to experience a sense of self-worth and prestige. If socially acceptable ways are unintersting or blocked, then alternative ways are found. One alternative is drugs: by means of drugs, one can improve one's moods, one can have better experiences, to the detriment of one's own body and at the expense of social risk (Wills 1985).

Thus, the structure of the entire network of social interaction and of communication processes via social values and goals is of fundamental importance. The adolescent's relationship to family, peers, school, work, and political as well as cultural areas will decide whether or not, and in what form, he or she will take drugs. Instability in the structure of his/her personality and low self-confidence are factors which promote drug consumption. Those adolescents with negative experiences and a low sense of integration as well as those who feel they have insufficient personal relationships are in danger of becoming drug consumers. They turn their backs on elementary norms of healthy behavior, and transgress legal norms in order to widen the horizon of their experiences (Silbereisen, Eyferth, & Rudinger 1986).

These findings are confirmed by the American longitudinal study by Jessor and Jessor (1977), who analyzed what they called "problem behavior" of a group of 12- and 13-year-olds and that of a group of 21- and 22-year-olds over a period of 10 years. The adolescents were questioned about behavioral and personality features and assessments of their social environment. In the area of personality variables and attitudes, problematic behavior goes hand in hand with a high sense of personal independence, a critical attitude towards social norms and values, low religious attachment, and a liberal attitude towards deviant behavior. According to Jessor and Jessor, the tendencies towards problem behavior are built on a personal pattern of attitudes which highly estimates unconventional behavior. Thus, it follows that the adolescents' desire for independence and more freedom, for more areas in which they can develop their competence, may be considered, on the whole, as a psychologically positive aspect.

However, behavior related to drug consumption clearly contains "regressive" elements, which show up as running away from problems, lack of flexible coping strategies, and a feeling of constraint. If adolescence is generally viewed as an attempt to establish a progression in life, in the course of which everything impersonal and normative is fought and pushed back, and where constraints through social codes of behavior, rigid moral outlooks, and conventional lifestyles are overthrown — in part only temporarily — then we have here the main motivational background for drug consumption. At the same time, according to Jessor and Jessor, this is an explanation for why illegal consumption of drugs is a form of behavior typical of the young, which diminishes quickly through increasing integration into various domains of adult life in the course of the third decade (Donovan & Jessor 1985).

Risk Constellations for Physical Diseases

The connection between an adolescent's physical complaints and his/her living conditions at school, at home, and in the leisure area were proven in studies undertaken by Engel and Hurrelmann (1988). These studies focus on information given by 13- to 16-year-olds concerning symptoms of health impairment. These symptoms are, for example, mentioned more frequently when there is a downward trend in school achievement. Adolescents who have repeated one or more classes or who have been forced to change schools because of poor performance complained much more frequently of headaches, strong heart beating, circulatory problems, stomachaches, etc. than other pupils. These adolescents are obviously aware of the risk of failure, with its long-term implications, and react to it with symptoms such as those mentioned above. These complaints are also mentioned more frequently when the adolescent attends a school which does not offer him or her a school-leaving certificate equal to that of his/her parents — expected social decline is "costly," and these costs may be of a physical or psychosomatic nature.

As this study shows, the values for psychosomatic complaints are especially high in those subgroups in which the pupil's academic record indicates that, with a high probability, he or she will not attain a level that will enable him or her to attain the parent's social status. This puts considerable stress on the pupil, which manifests itself in the form of psychosomatic complaints.

This study points out that failure in school, which carries the risk of occupational and social "downward mobility" in the future life course in comparison with the family of origin, can function as a social "stressor" which has detrimental effects on the social and emotional climate within the family and manifests itself in symptoms of psychosomatic and physiological disorders. The data support the hypothesis that psychosomatic symptom frequency is reinforced when adolescents experience failure in school and social and emotional conflict in their relationships with parents. Multivariate analysis shows that these effects are interconnected. Failure in school has a direct effect on the frequency of psychosomatic disorders, and an indirect effect by influencing social and emotional conflicts in the family. The underlying causes for the tensions between adolescents and their parents can be seen in the social and economic opportunity structures of the society (Hurrelmann, Engel, Nordlohne, & Holler 1988).

These data give evidence to the general assumptions of stress research stating that the manifestations of stress can be observed at many levels of the organism, including its psychological and emotional functioning, the nervous system, general physical health, and the functioning of various organs, as well as the endocrine and the immunological systems (Siddique & D'Arcey 1984; Pearlin 1987). Taking failure in school — or, more generally, the risk of downward mobility — as a "social stressor," and variants of the social and emotional family climate as "stress mediators," the study shows vegetative and physiological symptoms of psychosomatic disorders as "stress outcomes". The status insecurity resulting from failure in school can eventually be detrimental to health and well-being, particularly in cases where no favorable familial conditions exist that might lessen the impact of failure.

An adolescent can protect himself/herself to a certain degree from "reacting" with psychosomatic symptoms by dealing openly and actively with constellations of status insecurity. From studies in this area, we know that social networks with flexible and multiple forms of social support provide favorable impulses for an active style of coping with constellations of status insecurity (Gottlieb 1981). What must still be discovered is which specific structures and qualities of the social network heighten and which ones lower the risk of social dilemmas in adolescence as described above.

Stressors in Adulthood

We can distinguish two areas of living conditions in adulthood which have an effect on social and psychological disorders and health impairments:

1. Professional life, that is, the area where the individual is integrated into the domains of production and service in society
2. Family life and leisure time, that is, the individual's integration into nonprofessional forms of living and working — the reproductive domain of society

Both domains have an intense, mutual influence on each other. However, in all industrial societies, the specific conditions of work and professional life have an especially strong influence on the entire domain of the family and leisure.

In most population groups, the life expectancy has risen considerably, due to the constant improvement of working conditions, less hours of work per week, more vacation, improvements in housing conditions, effective sickness prevention, and better strategies for fighting illness and disease. For these reasons, the relationship between life and work has changed fundamentally. The individual's free time has increased. New possibilities for personal development (financial and temporal) concur with the temptations of mass consumption, leading to a disappearance of the contours of traditional forms of living and social-class milieus (Beck 1986, p.125).

As a result of this, the office and the factory have less importance for structuring the daily rhythms and patterns of life; the organization of the individual's private and leisure activities provide a multitude of possibilities and also require a great deal of energy and attention. On the other hand, the status of work is still extremely high, because social acceptance, social prestige, and the individual's financial status continue to depend on whether or not one is employed.

Several authors have argued that a process of "individualization" is typical for modern societies. Each person's life is pried free from prescribed norms, the course which his/her life will follow is open, depends upon individual decisions, and is a task which is squarely placed on each person's own shoulders (Elias 1987). Individualization, however, does not change the economic, political, and socially structured inequalities of life in modern societies. The high degree of individualization of daily life has turned into a structurally difficult starting basis in which the individual must establish his/her physical, psychological, and social identity. "Individualization" of lifestyles is accompanied by individual responsibility and accountability for the risks and failures which result thereof. For example, the social and economic processes which led to high unemployment are only indirectly seen as social problems — unemployment is seen, above all, as an individual problem and as a personal crisis which must be overcome with individual efforts. In modern society, there is as little security in employment and in different forms of work as there is in private/personal life, in parenthood, or in the relations with one's partner, lover, or spouse (Smelser & Erikson 1980; Elder 1985).

Modern societies place high demands on the individual's flexibility, and also on the stability of his/her capacities for self-regulation. Not every lifestyle which is socially possible is also beneficial physically or psychologically and vice versa: not every style of living which is satisfying physically or psychologically is socially acceptable. Moreover, the gap between how living conditions are conceptualized and how they are finally realized is increasing. Many individual concepts for living cannot be put into action because of concrete daily, structural demands and time-schedules imposed through work or lack of money. Each individual must try to find a balance, to make compromises, and to unify them in a way that promotes identity with his/her real concrete living conditions and personality structure (Sobel 1981).

In the following sections we will examine how demands of daily life and work, in the productive and reproductive sectors, affect social and psychological disorders and physical diseases in adulthood.

Professional Demands as Risk Factors

It has been shown that the individual's professional position — and thus his/her position in the social production processes — leads to different risks concerning mortality, morbidity, and the scope and degree of physical, psychological, and social deviation and disorder. Comparative studies have shown that members of working-class families had a much higher rate of morbidity (sicknesses per 100000 persons) and mortality (deaths per 100000 persons) than did members from middle-class families (white-collar employees, civil servants, owners of private businesses, etc.). Though the differences between the different professional groups have decreased in the last decades — confirming the tendency toward more equality of living and working conditions — they still exist today (Antonovsky 1979, p.100).

Statistics from different industrial nations prove that mortality is in inverse proportion to the prestige of the individual's professional group in society. Thus, studies made in Great Britain document a mortality rate in the lowest professional groups which is two and a half times greater than that of the top groups (Townsend & Davidson 1982). Other statistics show an inverse relation between the educational level — measured according to academic qualifications — and the probability of dying between 35 and 60 years of age. Those who completed university have the lowest probability, those with no school-leaving certificates whatsoever have the highest probability (Table 5).

The different mortality risks already begin at birth, and their effects become evident in infancy and childhood. The lower the social class from which the indi-

Table 5. Probability of death for men between age 35 and 60 according to selected professions, France, 1975–1980 (Oppolzer 1986, p. 31)

Professional group	Future life expectancy at 35 (in years)
Professors	43.2
Engineers	42.3
Self-employed	42.0
Teachers	41.1
Administrators	41.3
Technicians	40.3
Farmers	40.3
Managers from trade and industry	39.5
Small business owners	38.8
White-collar employees in trade	38.4
Office workers	38.5
Skilled workers	37.5
Household helpers	36.0
Unskilled workers	34.3
Average of all groups	38.8

vidual comes, the higher the rate of miscarriage, infant mortality, and child mortality (Oppolzer 1986, p.34). Due to improvements in hygiene and extended health care, the rate of infant mortality is declining in all population groups, but the social differences continue to exist (Townsend & Davidson 1982).

The main reason for the higher rates of morbidity and mortality among members of lower professional groups must be seen in the significant relationship between professional position (according to work and qualification) and the quality of living conditions, as they are influenced by the former. Disadvantages at work, unfavorable working conditions, and lower incomes usually lead to a disadvantage in material and housing conditions. For example, there are still fewer apartments available to the lower income groups than to those groups with higher incomes and better professions — on a quantitative level (number of rooms, persons per room, bedrooms for children) and on a qualitative level (toilet and bathroom facilities, central heating, garden, balcony, etc.). Usually, the social infrastructure (kindergartens, schools, services, etc.) is also inferior in the neighborhoods; environmental pollution (noise, air pollution) and traffic are greater. Therefore, the inequality in living conditions is still the main reason for unequal risks as far as morbidity and mortality are concerned (Kosa, Zola, & Antonovsky 1969).

Factors such as the professional position, economic and ecological factors (income, housing, work), as well as cultural and subcultural factors (educational training, leisure style, nutritional habits) definitely are significant for the genesis of psychological disorders and physical sicknesses. In an early study entitled *Mental Disorders in Urban Areas,* carried out in 1939, Faris and Dunham studied the distribution of patients who were mentally ill in the different social classes in greater Chicago by recording information concerning living and housing conditions in the different parts of the city, and combining this information with the number of recorded illnesses. The cases of mental illness were not equally distributed over the entire urban area, but, instead, were concentrated on the lower-class neighborhoods. In a similar study by Hollingshead and Redlich (1958), psychiatric patients from New Haven, Connecticut, were questioned about housing, income, profession, and education. Here, too, a clear overrepresentation of psychotic disorders in the lower classes was found. These tendencies are confirmed for physical diseases by newer studies. Most diseases, including infections, illnesses of the urogenital tract, illnesses of the digestive organs, heart/circulatory illnesses, and cancer are much more frequent in the lower social classes. These data show that the professional group to which one belongs influences a broad spectrum of conditions that are relevant to health (Kasl 1979; Cooper & Payne 1980).

Risk Factors Related to Work

What elements at work are most conducive to the individual's social, physical, and mental health, and which are least conducive? In a study carried out by Kornhauser (1965) on factory workers in Detroit, the following points were examined: safety conditions at work, physical working conditions, possibility of being creative on the job, repetition and machine rhythm, speed and intensity of work, social conditions and interactive embedding, status at work and possibility of working one's way up (getting ahead), forms of payment, and total income. Among the elements included by Kornhauser, the possibility of being creative turned out to be the most important factor; compared with this, factors like repetition and machine rhythm as well as speed and intensity of work were of little explanatory value. Subjectively perceived chances for getting ahead were also considered as being important.

Similarly, Kohn and Schooler (1983) found that "the fundamental complexity of work" was the decisive factor, defined as the degree to which the individual's own creative abilities and independent judgements are demanded. In detailed questions, information was gathered concerning the way in which the individual dealt with people, things, and data at work. It turned out that intellectual ability and the flexibility of imagination and creativity depended on the fundamental complexity of the work done: multiplicity of tasks, room for making decisions, varying psychological demands of the job, and relations with other people. The complexity of work correlates strongly with such factors as satisfaction with the job, feelings or self-worth, feeling competent, feeling depressed and having psychosomatic complaints, as well as the individual's general physical and mental health.

Conditions which are unfavorable for well-being are as follows: bad ergonomic working conditions (temperature, dust, light, noise), hard physical labor, monotonous, repetitive tasks which require little initiative, lack of social acknowledgement and lack of cooperation and communication at work, and the feeling of not being in control in respect to the situation at work. The more these factors are present in a job, the greater the general stress on the workers and the higher the probability that physical and psychological complaints will develop. It has been proved that combinations of physiological and psychological stressors are especially detrimental to health and well-being (Levi 1981).

Thus, tasks which require little initiative, a lack of cooperation, too little autonomy and self-determination, and a lack of insight into the general situation at work lead, in the long run, to disorders in the individual's well-being and to continuing physical and psychological complaints, to a breakdown of intellectual abilities and mental power, to passivity in the area of leisure, and to lack of engagement in politics; in other words, these factors influence one's entire lifestyle. There is a clear connection between the way in which an individual organizes his/her work, and the way in which he/she organizes the rest of his/her life. The human being's personality is mainly developed through coming to terms with his/her work, thus reflecting on all other areas of life (Kohn & Schooler 1983).

The new developments in technology have created new risks. Increasing anonymity and heterogeneity of social relationships can be among the social side effects of electronic-technical innovations (more automation, higher trends towards giant corporations, etc.). This leads to an increasing division of labor in many areas, with segmented tasks and social distance between colleagues.

Besides this, we still have the risks of the "old," traditional technologies at work. Use of different chemical and other toxic materials in mining, industry, and agriculture can lead to specific illnesses involving heart, lungs, bladder, and other types of cancer and illnesses caused by radiation. Reckless adherence to production methods which are particularly profitable can cause accidents at work, depression and alcoholism, as well as increased smoking, which, in turn, leads to bronchitis and lung cancer. Employing workers for tasks which are passive, repetitive, and mechanical can lead to psychosomatic and other stress-related illnesses. Environmental pollution affects large groups of the population (through lead poisoning or sulfur dioxide poisoning, etc.). Increased pressure to work more quickly leads to an increasing risk of accidents at work and in traffic. Pressure to use new energy sources which have not been adequately tested leads to health risks and fatalities, for example, through nuclear energy plants (House 1981; Frankenhaeuser 1981).

Unemployment as a Risk Factor

No matter how much unfavorable working conditions affect the individual's health, unemployment remains considerably more stressful than bad working conditions. In a study carried out in 1933 on unemployed people in Marienthal, the authors Jahoda, Lazarsfeld, and Zeisel tried for the first time to analyze exhaustively the social, psychological, and physical health effects of the phenomenon "unemployment." The authors describe four "types of attitudes" developed by the interviewees for coping with unemployment, or as a reaction to unemployment: optimistic, resigned, desperate, or apathetic. These attitudes are closely related to the individual's financial situation — those who are optimistic have the highest income, those who are apathetic the lowest. This relationship also applies to the health of the children involved: In the group of children with the best health, 38% of the fathers were working, in the group of children with the poorest health, none of the fathers were working (Jahoda, Lazarsfeld, & Zeisel 1971).

The social, psychological, and physical correlates of unemployment can only be understood in view of the losses which unemployment brings with it, even in today's changing relationship between life and work (Kasl, Gore, & Cobb 1975):

1. The day is no longer structured by work
2. Loss of financial security and the ability to satisfy material needs through money
3. Loss of new vistas which are related to work (individually in the from of a career, socially in the form of acknowledgement)
4. Loss of social contacts with colleagues
5. Loss of the ability to express oneself through work
6. Loss of the possibility for satisfying one's need to be productive
7. Loss of one's sense of importance in society
8. Loss of stimulation through the social environment
9. Loss of the role as wage earner and provider for the family

A survey of recent studies shows that unemployment results in an enormous increase in stress on the individual in question (Fagin 1985; Waller 1985, p.57). Even the announcement of planned shutdowns can lead to massive psychosomatic complaints and health impairment of the employees and their families. In case of long periods of unemployment, the risk of health problems becomes very high: heart disease, high blood pressure, and digestive disorders are in the forefront of illnesses related to unemployment. Furthermore, there is a marked increase in psychiatrically diagnosable illnesses and delinquency and in the suicide rate.

Stressful Events in Life Transitions as Risk Factors

As we have already discussed with a focus on childhood, psychological researchers have developed differentiated methods for recording an accumulation of "stressful life events." Holmes and Rahe (1967), for example, confront their interviewees with a list of life-changing events which all require the individual to (re)adjust socially. The interviewees themselves indicate the degree of stress involved for each event; that is, they are asked to estimate how much energy and time they would require to adjust to each specific event in the area of family constellations, marriage, financial stiuation and housing, relationships with the peer group, work, religious education, leisure time, and daily life. The Social Readjustment Rating Scale (SRRS) consists of a total of 43 life events including the following:

1. Death of spouse
2. Divorce
3. Separation from spouse
4. Imprisonment
5. Death of a family member
6. Hurting oneself or becoming ill
7. Marriage
8. Becoming unemployed
9. Reconciliation with one's spouse
10. Going into retirement
11. Changes in the health of a family member
12. Pregnancy
13. Sexual problems
14. Birth of a child
15. Occupational changes
16. Considerable changes in income
17. Death of a close friend

All of the events listed have one thing in common, namely that they require, as a rule, that the individual make a certain amount of effort to adjust and to cope. Many studies were able to provide empirical proof of a relationship between an accumulation of stressful events in life and psychological or physical disorders and illnesses. The relationship becomes especially intense when the spectrum of stress not only comprises unique stressful life events, but also life changes, life transitions and, especially, chronic stress (Rabkin & Struening 1976; Thoits 1983; Kessler, Price, & Wortman 1985).

Obviously, not only the immediate, dramatic challenges to the individual's ability to adjust are stressful, but also, and especially, the long-term consequences of unhappy love relationships, tension with one's children, tension with one's boss, chronic situations at work in which too many or too few demands are made, long-term financial problems, etc. All of these problems can exceed a person's capacity and can lead to depression, aggression, psychosomatic complaints, and alcoholism (Pearlin 1983; Pearlin & Lieberman 1979). It is harder to record these continuing stressful events than the current, "critical" ones. One promising method is to ask about daily problems and hassles which are viewed as difficult and bothersome, and behind which extreme chronic stress is sometimes hidden (Lazarus & Folkman 1984).

All pertinent studies provide proof that, in respect to stressful life events, the socially underprivileged groups show more symptoms of stress than other groups. It seems as if not only the stress components in underprivileged groups are not only objectively higher, but also the stress which is perceived subjectively. Furthermore, a feeling of not being able to cope with the daily challenges and developments of life is more prevalent in underprivileged groups, with the result that they often feel powerless against the demands which life makes on them; in addition, they are lacking in self-confidence, and often develop unsuitable strategies for coping (Albee 1987).

Due to concrete living situations, the underprivileged must cope with more stressful events and situations, and, at the same time, they are also more "vulnerable" to these concrete problems than people from the middle or upper classes. Kobasa (1979) and Kessler and Cleary (1980) explain this through the relatively limited access to psychological as well as to social resources, in other words, to the coping mechanisms and control techniques of living situations, on the one hand, and the material and nonmaterial support networks on the other.

These features of lifestyles are expressed through different social definitions of health and illness. People from the lower classes often view illness as a type of weakness which impairs or hinders the body's physical functioning. Illness is only then taken seriously when it can no longer be ignored. It seems as if physical sensations and symptoms which signal illness are simply not perceived as long as the pain involved is still bearable. This is why people from the lower classes consult doctors less often than do people from the upper or middle classes, even when the state of their health is poorer. People from the higher classes clearly take more advantage of preventive medicine and consult doctors more frequently for prophylactic reasons, all this with a view toward long-term "fitness" (Kosa, Zola, & Antonovsky 1969; Mechanic 1982).

Different concepts of health are also reflected in eating habits. In the lower classes, food which is considered to be especially nutritional and strengthening is preferred, whereas people from the higher classes prefer food which is easily digestible and natural. Furthermore, people from the middle and upper classes are more informed about healthy nutrition, and they keep up with the latest dietary findings.

As Bourdieu's analyses (1984) have shown, differences exist not only concerning food consumption and preparation, but also in eating and drinking habits. These differences can also be seen in body language and body control: People from the higher classes are more involved in and spend more of their free time on sports. It is easy for these classes to find a means of self-expression in sports, because they can bring their own values, which they develop through their own specific way of coping, into their sports activities: independence, responsibility for themselves, the desire to perform well, self-discipline, perseverance, motivation to succeed, and willingness to take specific risks.

As these findings have shown, all of the following points are deeply anchored in social structures: the individual's personal style of coping in all areas of daily life, including nutrition, behavior concerning drugs, physical and athletic activities, sleep, daily biological rhythm, working habits, leisure and relaxation and reproduction. The degree to which these forms of behavior are conducive to health, or harmful to it, differs. These forms of behavior can themselves be risk factors for various complaints and illnesses. Depending on one's situation in life, one will emphasize a certain relationship to one's body, a certain way of using the body, a moral and/or esthetic standardization of behavior, and an activation of certain norms oriented towards hygiene.

Chapter 4 Resources: Personal and Social Coping Capacities

As shown in the previous chapter, social, psychological, and physical stressors do not show up in symptoms of disorder in a monocausal, mechanical way. The resources that are available to an individual through his/her own efforts or in the form of support from the social environment determine the extent to which stressors take effect as potential risk factors.

The following description differentiates between:

1. Personal resources, which refer to the personal strategies of coping with stressful life-events, social role conflicts in the areas of education, work, partnership, and leisure, as well as to the individual capacity for action in dealing with transitions in the life course
2. Social resources, which refer to the various forms of support inherent in the social environment and in the network of social relationships which a person has access to, or that he/she can mobilize in difficult situations during the life course

Personal and social resources form and influence each other reciprocally to some extent. Together they constitute the capacity which a person has at his/her disposal for coping with life-events.

Personal Resources

Whether or not a stressful event or situation exceeds social, psychological, and physical adaptability is essentially determined by a person's behavioral capacities and action competencies. If, over a long period of time, a discrepancy exists between the demands on action within a particular sphere of life and a person's behavioral capacities, the risk of disorders and impairments is greatly increased.

Behavioral skills and capabilities — especially those which are essential for interaction and communication — are important prerequisites in a person's attempts to maintain and integrate his/her own motives, desires, and interests while adapting to the demands and requirements of the environment. Adaptation is an active process that is aimed in two directions, internally and externally. During the development of personality, behavioral competency is established for coping with internal and external reality, whereby a state of tension exists between both of these spheres.

In order to process internal and external reality, certain basic skills and abilities are essential. Each act of interaction with internal and external reality alters these skills and abilities, while at the same time contributing to their further development. The use of the term "processing" implies a "working on one's self," whereby an attempt is made to integrate impressions and experiences with previous knowledge, information, experiences, and observations (Hurrelmann 1988).

The term "action competency" is used to describe an individual's capacities in regard to the accessibility and use of skills and abilities for coping with internal and external reality. The development of such basic skills and abilities, which enable an individual to perceive and assimilate the social and objective-material environment with all of his/her senses, is a prerequisite for establishing behavioral competency. These basic skills and abilities include various aspects: sensory (e.g., taste, vision), motoric (e.g., physical mobility), interactive (e.g., ability to assume contrasting perspectives, willingness to make contact), intellectual (e.g., the ability to process information, capacity for storing knowledge), and emotional (e.g., ability to experience emotions, social ties, empathy). Such basic capacities are usually developed within the first few years of life (Hurrelmann 1988, p.157).

This process of developing basic skills and abilities, which is assisted not only by interorganismic processes of maturation, but also by stimulation from the social and material environment, leads to the establishment of behavioral competence: As soon as the sensory, motoric, interactive, intellectual, and affective skills and abilities are sufficiently differentiated and complex that an autonomous self-guided interaction and communication exists, action competence has been established. It describes the potential available and applicable at a particular stage of life in respect to awareness of the environment, bodily movements adequate to the prevailing physical and environmental conditions, the control of actions according to ethical and moral principles, the assimilation of the social and material environment appropriate to emotional needs, the pursuit of pleasure, the verbal naming and coding of external reality, as well as the ability to make social contact and to become self-confident in one's actions (Clausen 1986b).

The efficiency of the physiological systems (in particular, the central nervous systems, the cardiopulmonary systems, the muscle, ligament, tendon, and skeletal systems), and the composition and proportions of the body characterize the physical basis of each action. This basis must be viewed within a social and psychological context. In addition, motor-coordinating abilities which affect the quality of movement, the control of balance and reactions, the regulation of body rhythms, spatial orientation, versatility, and manual dexterity should also be included in the analysis, as well as measures of physical prowess such as the availability and mobilization of energy reserves, endurance, control of strength, mobility, and speed. To accomplish this will necessitate combining biological, medical, psychological, and sociological theories and research (Featherman & Lerner 1985; Baltes, Featherman, & Lerner 1986).

Capacities of Processing and Coping

Capacities of processing are an integral part of action competence. From the point of view of action theory, a person's behavior is based on a subjective representation of the environment. When carrying out an action, each individual adheres to a cognitive representation of the social and material reality. This image can be described as an inner model of external reality. Stored within this model are the environmental conditions which an individual regards as being important: knowledge of one's self and possibilities for action, and the expected course of action with its potential variations and consequences.

The security with which a person is able to function socially depends on the completeness and clarity of this model, and on its transposition into plans of action. If the goals are unclear, or if the knowledge of the consistency of one's own or other people's actions is inadequate, one lacks strategies suitable for transposing goals into actions, as well as criteria necessary for perceiving feedback. This can result in inaccurate perception of the prerequisites for one's own actions and inadequate information in respect to the goal of action, the assessment of the conditions underlying action, and the appraisal of feedback on one's own behavior. In addition, the execution of action can be impeded due to a lack of skills or to an inability to use them, or as a result of a lack of flexibility in carrying out such actions. Such inflexibility can be manifest in behavior which is rigid, stereotyped, or dictated by extreme social conformity. All of these factors prevent an adequate response to the immediate demands of a situation (Bandura 1977; Magnusson & Allen 1983).

As a rule, in approaching the specific demands of a particular social situation, individuals are equipped with a well-established program of possible responses, a particular level of knowledge, and numerous memories of previous experiences, all of which combine to form a particular style of behavior in dealing with new experiences. Each new event or situation represents an item of information that demands a particular behavioral response.

Reacting to a social situation in a competent manner necessitates utilizing various hierarchically structured phases of cognitive processing. This process usually takes place unconsciously, and only becomes conscious if an extremely novel or complex and demanding task arises, or if the social environment compels a person to reflect on his/her own reactions. If the processing of reality is carried out efficiently and accurately, prerequisites are established that enable the person to react to a situation in an adequate manner. If, within one or more of the stages, the processing is carried out in an inappropriate and inadequate manner, the likelihood of responding incompetently is increased (Dodge 1986).

The inability to process information completely and precisely can result in incompetent behavior. A disturbance in the person's system of information processing can take place when for some reason a step is inaccessible or is carried out in a distorted and one-sided manner, for example, when the basis of some information proves to be completely inadequate, or when the situation is interpreted incorrectly. Accordingly, distortion or deficiencies during the stages of processing can be causal factors in problem behavior (Dodge 1986).

Each individual has specific physiological and psychological prerequisites that have evolved in the course of his/her lifetime and that enable him/her to carry out information processes and to apply behavioral options. The ability to confront stressful events and situations competently is dependent on specific personality traits and on psychological processing variables whose individual form functions as a moderator between objective difficulties and subjective behavioral responses. Ulich (1987, pp.147–150) describes some of the important information-processing variables:

1. The Awareness Orientation. This represents the actualization of psychic energy. Experiencing and acting depend essentially on which aspects of the person-environment relationship receive attention during the act of perceiving. It appears that a high degree of self-awareness leads persons to pay greater attention to physical and psychological reactions when confronted with critical life-events and to plan and undertake corrective measures at an earlier point in time; this in turn results in their being less susceptible to deviance and disease.
2. Self-esteem. Various forms of self-esteem play a decisive role in the process of assessing the relative danger of a particular situation, in dealing with difficulties, and in the extent to which a crisis affects the future development of personality. The negative effect of continuous stress and critical life-events may result from the fact that such events lead one to develop a negative view of oneself. Restrictions are experienced in self-development, the satisfaction of basic needs, self-assertion and perseverance, and in the potential to organize one's life. Self-assessment and self-esteem can be influential in augmenting or diminishing the effects of external influences and crises on psychological health.
3. Confidence in Locus of Control. This variable is formed within the process of coming to a decision in respect to the extent that one feels able to anticipate a particular situation or its consequences, or to the extent that one feels able to influence or at least interpret them adequately. Here we are dealing with the cognitive realization of wishes, conceptions, and chances of success in regard to one's own capacity of influence.
4. Causal Attribution. This refers to a person's attempt to explain causality in environmental events. These subjective interpretations are not only manifestations of norms and previous experiences; they also process immediate impressions concerning the causes of problems and the possible causes of desired or undesired changes in one's own situation or state of mind.

All of these variables are inherent in the global processes of the appraisal of the type of difficulty (threat, challenge, injury/loss) and the degree of stress which a situation generates. This appraisal determines to some extent whether an event, a problem, or a situation is regarded as being relevant to one's desires or aims, whether one feels capable of defending oneself, and which kind of coping strategy can be mobilized and applied. Cognitive and emotional appraisal is generally multidimensional and specific to a particular area; it must be differentiated into various subprocesses that do not always run parallel to one another and that do not always result in a uniform judgement in respect to potential threats and relevant coping strategies (Lazarus & Folkman 1984).

The individual's coping capacity is determined by the adaptability to specific stressors such as, for example, critical life-events. Where such events are regarded as being threatening or injurious — inasmuch as they overtax one's capabilities of responding to and overcoming such difficulties — the risk increases that stress symptoms and ensuing psychological and organic disorders may occur. As a result, stress is conceived of as being a process that contains cognitive as well as emotional and behavioral components. According to this concept, the cognitive appraisal of the external situation determines whether or not stress reactions occur, and what form these reactions will take. The term "stress" incorporates confrontations with injury, loss, threats, and challenges of various kinds, to the extent that the well-being of the person is affected and his/her coping strategies are overtaxed and exhausted (Lazarus & Folkman 1984).

According to this action-theory concept, stress occurs when a person experiences a discrepancy between demands, challenges, and the available coping strategies, while at the same time experiencing the discrepancy and its potential consequences as a threat. If, after appraisal of the causes and effects of the strain, on the one hand, and of the individual action competences, on the other, the coping strategies are judged to be adequate, the process of coping is terminated. If the capabilities are not sufficient, the individual experiences continuous strain that can lead to psychological, somatic, and psychosomatic symptoms; these, in turn, affect the individual coping strategies. Ultimately, the attempt to resolve the difficulties leads to a reappraisal of the stressful event. If the coping strategies are adequate, the stress is overcome; if they prove inadequate, the stress is experienced as a continuous crisis.

Recent theoretical approaches attempt to integrate the stress paradigm more systematically into a social and socioecological context (Kessler, Price, & Wortman 1985). In this understanding, the term "stress" depicts a person's inability to deal with the discrepancy between his/her desires and needs, and the existing social circumstances which are preventing their fulfillment.

This broad definition of the term "stress" has also been incorporated into social psychological research. In addition to the role played by the quantity of stressful events measured, one has come to realize the subjective importance of such events and their consequences for a person's concept of self and of external reality. This direction of research confirms that stress, in addition to its objective influence (e.g., overtaxing work situations due to shortage of time) also has a subjective importance (e.g., in the perception or appraisal of a situation). This is especially noticeable where a substantial discrepancy exists between the objective difficulties and the subjective coping strategies.

Different Styles of Processing and Coping

Generally speaking, factors such as confidence in one's emotional stability, the ability to solve problems, social skills that enable one to approach others for support and help, and stable self-esteem and sense of identity can be regarded as being favorable prerequisites for a successful confrontation with internal and external stressors. Each individual has access to a particular basic pattern of reacting to and coping with reality. This basis allows for a habitual and consistent pattern of behavior over diverse situations, and enables a person to master environmental as well as internal demands, and to resolve conflicts between these demands (Lerner 1976; Murphy & Moriarty 1976; Pearlin & Schooler 1978; Werner & Smith 1982).

This pattern of coping strategies is especially effective if mobilized before the occurrence of the stressful event, or at least before the manifestation of the first symptoms of stress. Such an anticipatory problem-solving behavior assumes a special role in coping processes, essentially because it enables the individual to select situations, to choose his/her own behavioral potential in accordance with particular situations, and, as a consequence, actively shape the challenging situation. In complex situations of a stressful nature which are already manifest and as such cannot be easily altered, anticipatory coping is doubtlessly more effective than the mobilization of any form of defensive, reactive, or suppressive behavior.

Empirically, the simplest form of measuring the extent and style of coping behavior is the use of self-report questionnaires. In the area of scholastic achievement, for example, one can develop a questionnaire describing a situation in which the students are asked to imagine that they have just experienced failure in scholastic performance. The anticipatory coping attempts can be characterized by statements such as the following: "I will attempt to find out what went wrong/I will improve my performance next time/I will get another chance/I will attempt to seek some assistance." The defensive/projective coping pattern can be characterized by statements such as the following: "In my opinion, the test was unfair/The teacher is to blame/I am angry at the teacher/I am angry at the others." The suppressive coping attempts are characterized by statements such as the following: "It doesn't bother me/I try to forget that I failed/I just don't look at the results/I just don't think about it afterwards." Similar constructions can be developed for other areas and other populations (Schwarzer 1985).

An empirical examination based on questionnaires must be supplemented by interviews and observations that are directed towards a detailed reconstruction of the individual's previous history of problem-solving behavior. However, the single measurement of the strength of various forms of coping behavior must not be regarded as a stable personality trait that exists independently of concrete social situations, but as behavior that is socially learned and regulated by cultural factors. Such studies can only be used as a general guide to habitual coping strategies and processing attempts that are connected to the social organization of life in general.

When regarding the individual's coping capacity, a distinction can be made between two separate concepts: inadequacy resulting from a lack of competence (competence deficit), and inadequacy resulting from a failure to utilize existing skills (competence disorder). A competence disorder exists when a person is confronted with a challenge for which he/she has not yet developed suitable coping strategies with which to master the challenge adequately. This situation can occur, above all, when a person is confronted with new life-events, or when he/she enters a new phase of life. A situation in which skills are available but are not implemented or only partially utilized can be expected to arise when abilities that have already been learned have not been sufficiently integrated to allow for their deployment in situations that differ greatly from the situations in which they were originally acquired. In addition, competence can be impeded because existing skills are prevented from being applied due to psychological barriers, social insecurity, or ambiguous role definitions (Lauth 1983, p.20).

Processing capacities and coping strategies have a substantial effect on physical, psychological, and social well-being, because they act as moderating factors. However, they reach the limits of their influence when difficulties arise that are connected with conditions inherent in the prevailing social structures, and that cannot be influenced by the individual: Even an anticipatory coping style is incapable of protecting the individual against the consequences of poverty, unemployment, or bad working conditions. Such consequences cannot be changed or mastered by a single individual. In such situations, only collective strategies can be expected to bring success (Pearlin 1987). This aspect will be examined again while reviewing social resources.

Gender-Specific Styles of Processing and Coping

The analysis of processing and coping styles has brought forth numerous indications of gender-specific qualities. In Chapter 2 it has already been shown that, in comparison with males, the prevalence of delinquent and criminal acts among females is extremely low. We have here an interesting case of differing reactions to similar if not identical conditions. Disturbed family relationships, an unfavorable social climate within the family, punitive child-rearing methods, material deprivation, criminal history on the part of the parents, and other such social risk factors evidently do not lead to a prevalence of delinquency or behavioral disorders on the part of young females that is anywhere near that of young males. In particular, the number of females involved in acts of violent crime and other forms of aggressive delinquent behavior is extremely low (Rutter 1980). The number of females involved in traffic offences is also extremely low. Despite the large increase in the proportion of women drivers within the last few years, behavior patterns in this area seem to be present which result in the high degree of gender-specific social conformity, integration, and sense of responsibility typical of women (Keupp 1982).

The socialization of females evidently limits their proneness to problem behavior of an antisocial and aggressive nature at a very early stage in life. Delinquent behavior, as an expression of attempts at coping with situations and conflicts, must be regarded as being the result of a social learning process by which, in comparison with males, females resort less to aggressive and destructive patterns of behavior, and in which they are less likely to transform their aggression into actions directed towards the social and physical environment. Due to a social learning process, when compared with men, women show more of a tendency to resolve tension and conflicts through internal intrapsychic processes. At the same time, women have access to a wide spectrum of forms of deviant behavior that are tolerated by society. These forms include the high rate of attempted suicide among women, the phenomenon of the problem drinker as a typically female form of alcoholism, the prevalence of psychosomatic symptoms and neurotic illness, the phenomenon of reactive depression and the high degree of physical ailments. It is important to note that, in addition to their appellative nature, all of these symptoms have an indirect and subtle aggressive component that can, for example, take the form of revenge or accusations of guilt directed towards the social environment. The greater part of disturbed social behavior among females appears to be essentially a reaction to real or assumed conflicts in personal relations (Keupp 1982, p.227).

In fact, as already described, psychological and psychiatric studies of female adolescents that have been carried out since earliest childhood show more symptoms which are internally directed and withdrawn, such as neurotic behavior, anxiety, depression, and psychosomatic disorders. In contrast, male youths display a tendency towards acting-out and conflict-oriented disorders that are outwardly directed, such as aggression, drug abuse, and criminal behavior (Gove & Tudor 1973; Kessler & McLeod 1984; Gove 1985).

Both sexes presumably have specific, typical styles of expressing social and psychological strain that, in terms of personality dynamics, may be functionally equivalent. Whereas the male style is directed more towards acting-out behavior, the female style is more inwardly directed. These behavioral styles are intensified whenever an exaggerated fixation on the respective socially determined, gender-specific ideals can be observed. If, however, we consider the various forms of social, psychological, and somatic disturbances in their entirety, we find that the gender-specific differences are more or less neutralized.

Action Competencies During the Life Course

The capacity for mastering life-events has to be dynamically modified during the life course. Social and technological developments as well as psychological and physical changes demand a continuous adaptation of the behavioral repertoire and the capacities for coping and mastery in order to generate and coordinate adequate responses to environmental demands and to explore the possibilities within the social environment that contribute towards the development of abilities. This applies to the contribution made by the individual in respect to structuring situations, acquiring new ways of responding and coping, the continual scrutiny of existing forms of coping, and to the affective and emotional cathexis and incorporation of coping styles, as well as their integration into the self-concept.

Within each phase of life, competencies can be identified that are typical of a particular stage of development and that can be defined as being prerequisites and consequences for future stages of development. If, within one stage of life, the coordination and organization of personal resources is successfully accomplished, it can be expected that the individual will be able to cope adequately with future challenges: A competent individual is able to apply personal and environmental resources in such a way that a favorable basis for personal development ist established (Clausen 1986a, b).

Current thought in developmental research has seen the establishment of the term "developmental tasks" as an analytical concept which describes the transposition of society's demands into individual behavioral strategies. Developmental changes over the entire life course are examined within the context of concrete competencies which are necessary to deal with challenges in respect to various aspects of daily life. The development of this concept owes a great deal to the educational psychologist Havighurst (1956). According to this concept, physical, psychological, social, cultural, and moral development are viewed as being connected to a process of active learning extending over the entire life course, which is embedded in an environment that is regarded as being equally active.

According to Havinghurst's concept, developmental tasks vary in the degree to which they are dependent on culture and society. Some tasks, such as biological maturation, are of a universal nature and remain unchanged from culture to culture. Other tasks exist only within certain societies or within certain subcultures. The point in time at which the respective task is manifest and mastered is also an important aspect of development. Some tasks are limited in duration, whereas others encompass various dimensions and extend over several stages of life, such as, for example, the task of forming adequate relationships with peers of both sexes (Oerter & Montada 1987).

Obviously, the mastery of one developmental task, for example in the area of employment/occupation, affects the way in which confrontations in other areas take place, for example, in partnerships. According to this concept, developmental tasks do not exist in isolation; they can only be singled out for the purpose of analysis. In addition, developmental tasks must be viewed within the entirety of the historical context of their respective societes (Newman & Newman 1975).

With this model, developmental tasks can be described for various stages of life (Table 6).

In each of these life stages, a discrepancy can evolve between social, psychological, and physical demands, on the one hand, and one's capabilities, on the other, and which is then experienced as threatening or stressful. An examination of the distribution of symptoms of social deviation, psychological disturbances, and physical ailments within various stages of life reveals a certain discontinuity:

1. Disorders such as delinquency, criminal behavior, and the consumption of illegal substances are most prevalent in late adolescence. They are a typical expression of problems of social adaptation and integration.
2. The prevalence of various forms of psychological disturbance differs from one life phase to another. Hyperactivity is most prevalent in early childhood,

Table 6. Developmental coping capacities and developmental tasks during the life course

Phase of Life	Example of developmental behavior demands
Early childhood	Development of "basic trust" Formation of social ties Sensomotoric intelligence Preconceptual thinking Basic sensory and motor skills Symbolic and verbal expression
Late childhood	Ability to deal with peers Adequate gender-specific behavior Basic skills in reading, writing, and calculation Establishment of conscience, morals, and values Positive attitude to oneself as a growing organism
Early adolescence	Formal intellectual operations Scholastic achievement Establishment of relationships with both sexes Acquisition of male or female role Acceptance of own physical appearance Effective use of physical prowess
Late adolescence	Reappraisal of relationship to one's own body Abstract intellectual operations Emotional independence from parents and other adults Preparation for marriage and family life Preparation for an occupation System of values that serve as a guideline for behavior Stabile self-image and sense of identity Use of consumer market
Early adulthood	Choice of partner Foundation of a partnership with a member of the opposite sex Entry into field of employment Establishment, support, and care of a family Organizing a household Responsibility as a citizen Childbirth Development of an individual lifestyle
Advanced adulthood	Separation from one's own children Reinforcement and continual redefinition of partnership Responsibility as a citizen Consolidation or reappraisal of occupational career Directing of energies towards new roles and tasks
Old age	Acceptance of one's own life Ability to adapt to reduction in physical strength Development of an attitude towards death

whereas learning difficulties are encountered mostly in late childhood and early adolescence. The frequency of suicide attempts and particular disturbances such as anorexa nervosa is highest in late adolescence, whereas depression, neurotic, and psychotic disturbances are most prevalent in adulthood, and to some extent in old age.

3. Physical diseases are most prevalent in the postnatal stage, remain at a low level in adolescence and early adulthood, and are a typical phenomenon which occurs with greater frequency among older adults.

Presumably, in each stage of life particular developmental and age-related forms of productive as well as unproductive coping strategies emerge that are directed towards internal and external reality whenever adaptability is overtaxed. In adolescence, those forms of irregular behavior are most prevalent that symbolize a rebellion against the social order and social structure of the adult world, whereas during childhood, disorders of a biological-organic nature prevail. In adulthood, additional disorders come to the fore that result from maladaptivity and inadequacies that can be traced back to limitations on the capacities of psychological and physical energy.

Social Resources

In addition to personal resources, social resources must be examined in their capacity as mediating and moderating forces in dealing with various stressors in the life course. Whether the social, psychological, and physical adaptability is over-taxed, and how this affects further personality development is determined essentially by the amount of support contained in a person's social environment and in the structure of the social network into which he/she is integrated.

The Importance of Social Ties

In studies undertaken at the beginning of this century, Emile Durkheim drew attention to a relationship between suicide and a lack of social integration, which was especially apparent in the context of old age, and psychological health. Whereas the "anomic" suicide has its roots in a deficit in socially regulative mechanisms, the "egoistical" suicide was regarded as being the result of a deficit in social ties of a religious and personal nature. Just as the directive influence of religion, especially Catholicism with its strong internal bonds and practical guidance, served to contribute towards the mastery of critical life-events, Durkheim regarded the social relationships which are inherent in the family as having a similar effect. Married persons were seen to have a greater "immunity" and to generally possess a better "psychological and moral constitution" compared with unmarried individuals; when marriage and the home were intact, a crisis could be dealt with more easily (Durkheim 1951). Durkheim regarded the protective effect of social relationships to be the result of a structural "embedment". The factors important to the phenomena of suicide were the density of the family, defined as the number of children, and the symmetry of the relationship between the spouses.

Although recent studies have failed to support these findings in every detail, Durkheim must be given credit for having in the first place drawn attention to the "protective function" of social ties in confrontations with stressful life-events. Current studies seem to confirm his basic premises.

An investigation by Berkman and Breslow (1983) in the San Francisco area, for example, showed a relationship between health-relevant behavior and the integration into a matrimonial style of partnership or a parent-child relationship. The existence of a well-functioning matrimonial relationship proved to be one of the most favorable factors in the maintenance of well-being and health. Such a partnership is evidently a good prerequisite for personality development; it reduces the danger of psychological disorders, aggressive and delinquent behavior, and increases the willingness to receive medical or psychiatric treatment should disorders or impediments occur. The mortality and morbidity rates of married adults are considerably lower than those of divorced or single adults.

The author's explanation of these findings is essentially based on the importance that social ties have on behavior. The existence of a close personal relationship evidently has a disciplining and controlling effect on behavior in general, and at the same time fosters behavior which is conducive to good health. Such behavior is affected directly through the internalization of norms for responsible behavior, and, indirectly, through the controlling influence which one's partner exerts through regulation and stimulation. Consequently, the existence of closely knit, stable social ties functions as a social control. Physical and psychological health is therefore maintained through the suppression of deviant and unconventional behavior, and through the encouragement of such behavior as sports activities, low consumption or abstinence from tobacco, weight control, little or no alcohol usage, regular sleeping habits, and the adherence to medical treatment — all of which are more likely to be observed in well-functioning partnerships (Leavy 1983).

Thoits (1983) addresses the importance of the stability of social support. Stressful events evidently have less effect on symptoms of disorder when, over a long period of time, an individual has had access to a high degree of social support which is structurally secure, stabile, and dependable. The variety of modes of support within the social network proves to be extremely important. Research findings show that in a stressful situation it is especially favorable when a person can fall back on more than one form of social support, and when the communication between the various peers and peer groups is good (Kahn & Antonucci 1980).

The research in this area to date has been reviewed by Gottlieb (1983) and Keupp and Röhrle (1987). Most of the studies show evidence for Durkheim's proposition that the extent and quality of social relationships have an effect on health. The more subjectively satisfactory and objectively helpful an individual's personal and social networks are, the smaller the probability of psychological and/or somatic complaints. Most researchers regard social support as a "buffer" between stressful life-events and other risk factors, on the one hand, and the social, psychological, and physical symptoms of disturbance and impairment, on the other.

The Concept of a "Social Network"

The central idea of these studies stems from the research into social "networks" and can be expressed as follows: The more a person is integrated into a network of social relationships, the more he/she is able to cope with unfavorable living conditions, critical life-events, and long-lasting, stressful situations, and the less likely it is that symptoms of stress such as social, psychological, and physical disorders will emerge. In other words, a social network of relationships is regarded as having a supportive function when a person is exposed to stressors.

A social network is often referred to as a "social immune system," in analogy to biological systems of protection and immunity. Cassel (1975), for example, regards biologically protective factors as being an organism's process of adaptability to changes in the environment. He views psychosocial protective factors as being the form and strength of group support that is available to an individual. The presence of members of a primary group provides for the satisfaction of those needs for integration and a sense of belonging, which, under the conditions of present-day society, are being increasingly jeopardized, and whose continuing neglect can lead to deficits in psychological functioning, lead to impairment of the nervous system and hormone balance, and probably contribute to the emergence of chronic illnesses. Both biological and social protective factors have a buffering effect when an individual is confronted with difficulties.

In order to contribute towards more precision and transparence in examining supportive relationships, it is necessary to differentiate between the terms "social network" and "social support" (Cobb 1976; Heller & Swindle 1983). A social network refers to a web of social relationships which a person is bound into. The network consists of the sum of the contacts that a person has with other individuals. It can be described and analyzed according to various criteria, and its support potential is determined by the characteristics of the structure, the quality and the function of the relationships within the network. We must examine which aspects of a person's network of social contacts and relationships can actually be termed supportive, and which of these aspects are perhaps nonsupportive or even detrimental.

Presently, various empirical instruments exist that can identify members within the social network, and their function as providers of social support. Instruments have also been developed that attempt to measure the various kinds of social support that a person perceives and experiences. However, the theoretical and methodological verification of these instruments is not yet completely satisfactory. As a rule, social support is measured retrospectively, that is, after a problem has arisen. This process can, of course, be affected by distortion, errors, lapses in memory, and by a cognitive reappraisal of the events and their consequences (Leavy 1983).

Questionnaires that measure social support generally consist of simple questions based on sociometric considerations (e.g., Sarason, Levine, Basham, & Sarason 1983; Schwarzer 1985). The salient items are as follows:

1. Who listens to you when you have a desire to talk to someone?
2. On whom can you depend when you experience a crisis, even when it means inconveniencing the person?
3. Whom can you really rely on when you need help?
4. Which person accepts you completely with all your good and bad sides?
5. Which person is able to comfort you when you are suffering from stress and strain?

With this method, which, if possible, should be enhanced with interviews and long-term observations, one can achieve a rough estimate of a person's potential support network. In most versions of such questionnaires an attempt is made to determine how satisfied the person is with the support received by the persons named. Other instruments of measurement form indexes that give information about the instrumental and affective contribution of social support; they also differentiate between the social support available, and that which is experienced and described (Schwarzer 1985).

Characteristics of Support Networks

Social support stems from various key persons who are members of a network. As a rule, empirical studies distinguish between the following groups of reference persons: parents, brothers and sisters, friends, colleagues, relatives, teachers, superiors, and persons in an advisory and assisting capacity. The effective degree of socioemotional or instrumental help varies according to the key persons and key groups.

Research literature classifies the various degrees of closeness and integration within networks of relationships into three categories:

1. Confidant Relationships. A confidant is a person with whom one can discuss the most intimate problems, whom one can trust, and whose help can be elicited at all times. One's parents, friends, spouses, brothers, sisters, and children are probably the most likely candidates to be a confidant.
2. Closely Knit Relationships. The relationship's degree of closeness and intimacy can be determined by the frequency of interactions and the resulting probability of common values and interests. It can also be determined by the intensity of mutual feelings of good will or social respect based on common experiences and events of a formative nature that may have taken place at a much earlier date. Mainly, family members and friends are potential candidates for close relationships.
3. Loosely Knit Relationships. These are relationships of a more superficial nature in which mutual obligations are minimal. The duration of such a

relationship may be short, and its content may be characterized through the absence of emotional ties. Nevertheless, the persons involved are familiar with and respect each other. The framework of such relationships is usually found in factors that are common to both parties, such as: fields of employment, areas of residency, leisure time interests, membership in organizations, clubs, religious, or political groups (Badura 1981, p.36).

Social support can be regarded as an interpersonal transaction that takes place in various dimensions. The support potential of a social network consists of continual or intermittent activities on the part of other persons that contribute to an individual's stability and provide feedback about his/her own and other people's actions, and that assist in overcoming situations of deprivation and stress (Cobb 1976; Gottlieb 1981; Kessler & McLeod 1985).

The structural characteristics of the support network have an important effect on the forms and dimensions of support. Within networks, the following structural characteristics play an important role:

1. Size: the number of individuals who are connected with each other
2. Density: the ratio of existing connections to potential connections
3. Frequency: the number of contacts per unit of time
4. Intensity: the importance of the content of the relationship for the person
5. Duration: the length of time that the relationship has existed
6. Direction: whether one-sided or reciprocal and symmetrical
7. Content: breadth of themes which can be discussed
8. Variation: combination of various kinds of social contacts and contents

From these structural characteristics one cannot make a direct assumption about the quality of support. The dimensions and the nature of the individual types of support also play a vital role. One can, in agreement with House (1981a), distinguish between emotional support (expressions of regard and acceptance), instrumental support (offers of financial assistance, concrete helping behavior), informative support (provide information and knowledge), and support in making judgements (offers to assess and solve problems).

Research to date shows that the size and density of a network are not necessarily advantageous in all dimensions. It is the functions and tasks which are in the foreground of an interaction that determine whether size and density have a positive effect. The strength of a closely knit network lies in the continuity of help available during long-term stress. The nuclear family is especially prominent as an aid to preventing and mastering difficulties. Friends and acquaintances appear to be important sources of information and support, whereby the main focus of their activity lies in short-term assistance and spontaneous help. Friends are not consciously defined as "helpers," which results in their help being especially effective. This is due to the absence of obligations and legitimate demands, and to the voluntary character of such help (Nestmann 1988). Also, relationships with neighbors can be regarded as being extremely important due to the access to a broad behavioral spectrum and to the degree of intimate knowledge inherent in such relationships. However, compared with friends and members of the family, we find that the kinds of help which are offered or solicited by neighbors are restricted in nature and only applicable to specific areas (Froland, Pancoast, Chapman, & Kimboko 1981).

The empirical studies show that the resources available in small, closely knit social networks are not of a unidimensional and homogeneous character, and are not continuously reciprocal; instead they often appear to be ambivalent and of a compulsive or coercive nature. Tensions and conflicts exist side by side with helping components. Dense and closely knit networks can also form a stable set of norms which are enforced by sanctioning individual members.

In contrast, within networks which are loosely knit and less intense, seeking help appears to be less influenced by the prevailing group norms. As the ties within such networks are less strong, their members often seek support in a broader spectrum of formal and informal resources. These loose ties can act as important sources of information and advice and enable individuals to look beyond the limitations inherent in close relationships. Consequently, in comparison with closely knit networks, such loose ties contain a greater potential for gaining knowledge and access to various sources of information and help. In novel situations and during the passage from one stage of life to another, relationships of this type encourage more adaptability and permit one to establish new contacts with friends and neighbours (Gottlieb 1983).

Support networks which are closely knit, small, dense, and have multiple functions are therefore especially dependable, and offer relatively comprehensive support in the face of difficult situations and continuous stress. On the other hand, they tend to be controlling, restrictive, normatively regulative, and therefore of an externally determined, involuntary nature. In comparison, broad, loosely knit relationships are open, potentially inspiring, have many stimulating facets, are self-regulatory, and usually voluntary. On the other hand, such relationships are less secure, are at greater risk, have first to be agreed upon, and when examined closely, tend to be limited in the breadth, intensity, and duration of the effectiveness of the support which they provide (Nestmann 1988, p.113).

Integration within a social network is essentially favorable to general well-being; however, it does not automatically guarantee that a suitable constellation of supporting factors will be mobilized under conditions of stress. Support which is inappropriately applied can have a negative effect, for example, when the help offered amplifies disturbed and distorted role behavior, when feelings of guilt and shame are increased because an individual is forced to depend on others and is not able to be supportive in return, when a person's self-concept of being a "failure" is inadvertently reinforced, or when false hopes and expectations are awakened in the face of difficulties which cannot be overcome. In this way, dependency can be created and reinforced, and the person in question can be maneuvered into role behavior which is characterized by helplessness and lack of initiative. In other words, social networks are not always helpful and supportive. They can also create conflicts and stress and have a detrimental effect, even when the motivation and willingness to help is present (Keupp & Röhrle 1987).

Mechanisms of Social Support

Generally speaking, the mechanisms by which social support is effective have not yet been sufficiently investigated. Two questions still open to debate are the extent to which social support can be predominantly traced back to the structural characteristics of the network and the extent to which the subjective view of those involved in the process of helping would be more likely to reveal information about the effect of support (the position held by most of the recent research). Future research must attempt to reconstruct in more detail those mechanisms that give answers to the question of why particular social conditions and/or social help have an effect on individual health. The main difficulty lies in understanding the complexity of the social, psychological, and somatic processes that are affected by these conditions.

Research to date points out three particular mechanisms of effect (Gottlieb 1981; Berkman 1985):

1. Social support can decrease the probability of stressful situations occurring; for example, good integration in social relationships produces a lesser degree of deficits of behavioral capacities and action competencies ("screening effect").
2. Social support can assist in coping with stressful situations where social and instrumental support are available that contribute towards competent processing of situations. In particular, support can increase a person's ability to withstand stressful situations before reacting with symptoms of stress, can strengthen self-esteem and a sense of control in stressful situations, and offer assistance that protects against despair and depression in the face of existing strain ("buffering effect").
3. Social support can directly affect the ability to deal with manifest symptoms of stress. For example, help and support can increase the ability to tolerate psychological and physical illness ("tolerance effect").

It is important to note different and manifold interdependencies: For example, difficult situations in the life course and life-events — such as the death of a near one, chronic illness, scholastic failure, regional mobility, etc. — can lead directly to changes in the social environment and to impairments in the support network. Conversely, behavioral disorders can lead to changes in a person's social network, for example, by causing isolation or stigmatization, and, as a consequence, add to the constellation of risk factors. On the other hand, during the process of coping with stress, the network of social support can undergo a process of intensification and expansion, for example, through self-help groups. Such reciprocal processes should be examined in more detail in future research (Leavy 1983; Seeman, Seeman, & Sayles 1985).

The support potential contained in the social network depends on the strategy of selection which a person employs. The social composition, size, and structure of the network is influenced to a great extent by the person's own activity. In other words, a person actively influences the social network's overall characteristics and its potential for support. Each individual can establish and modify supportive social networks of his/her own accord. Social support is not a static condition; it is a developing process that is influenced by prior supportive experiences and that adapts and changes in accordance with the effects of stressful events.

Social support, therefore, is not to be regarded as a fixed entity that is equally accessible to everyone; it must be apprehended and perceived by the individual. The patterns of reaction to risk factors in the life course, which are developed by a person during the life course, determine whether or not the search for social support among his/her confidants and reference persons becomes part of an effective coping strategy.

Chapter 5   Interdependencies: The Stress-Health Relationship

This chapter summarizes the foregoing discussion and presents explanatory models of the genesis and development of social, psychological, and somatic disorders and interrelates them. Instances of overlap and areas of convergence will be of particular interest because they indicate possible starting points for comprehensive interdisciplinary approaches. Although the different forms of disorders cannot be subsumed under one all-embracing theory, the general theoretical and methodological aspects they may have in common, and the actual connections between the various theories should be clearly identified in order to insure an efficient cooperation of the various scientific disciplines involved.

Traditionally, physical diseases have been explained in terms of organic factors, psychological disorders in terms of intrapersonal factors, and social deviance in terms of societal factors.

The "classical" approach of *medical science* to explaining illness, for example, rests on the assumption that any disorder has a specific cause, and can be traced back to a particular malfunction of the organism. It further assumes that any instance of ill health manifests typical external symptoms, and can therefore be diagnosed by scientifically trained experts. As a rule, an illness is thought to follow a certain course that can be described and predicted on the basis of known biological facts. In this sense, a symptom is an indicator that an organism or parts thereof do not function "normally," which means that they deviate from established standards. In this traditional medical model, normality and abnormality are clearly defined, separate states of the organism (cf. Engel 1962).

The traditional *psychological approach* to explaining psychological disorders starts from abnormal psychodynamic processes that are innate or have been acquired at an early stage of development, resulting from problems with the adjustment and coordination of needs, motives, and emotions, and leading to a subsequent malfunction of behavioral control. Such disorders are seen primarily to be rooted in intrapersonal tension and conflict, which have a detrimental effect on further personality development. The learning theoretical variant of this approach assumes that interferences or distortions affect the perception of impulses emanating from the environment, which leads to a construction of cognitive schemata that are inadequate for the processing of information (cf. Erikson 1959; Ulich 1987).

The traditional *sociological approach* concentrates on the political, social, and cultural structures as the prime causes of social deviance. In its simplest form, the approach assumes a malfunctioning — to use the concept of the medical model —

of the social and/or the value system, a disruption of elementary societal processes. This malfunctioning may produce strained social contacts and lead to individual behavior disorder and illness. Most variants of this model interpret illness as an outcome of social conditions, particularly of the conditions of production, class differences, and value and power structures. Accordingly, illness would be attributable, for example, to the individual's alienation from society, being largely the result of his or her lack of control over working conditions and social institutions (cf. Navarro 1976).

The three explanatory models outlined above are valid for the analysis of specific subject areas. On the other hand, they can only cover segments of reality. In isolated form, they analyze various aspects of the organism, individual, or environment. These must be integrated into a comprehensive model, if a framework for an interdisciplinary conception of a "healthy" personality development is to be arrived at. Thus, there should be less concentration on somatic, psychological, and social symptoms as separate categories. As has been pointed out in the previous chapter, personality, in all its functions and dimensions, does not develop independent of society, but is subject to the historically determined tension-field of social environment. Nor does personality evolve independent of concrete physical and psychological structures; it is always determined by biological and psychological factors.

During the last two decades, views and assumptions relating to normal and abnormal personality development have increasingly moved away from monocausal explanations and the underlying epistemological models of personality that one-sidedly focus on the organic, psychological, and social impulses of human development. The models that are now emerging are more differentiated; their main concern is for the interrelations between body, psyche, and environment (Goslin 1969; Baltes, Featherman, & Lerner 1986; Clausen 1986b).

The scientific discussion of these problems is facilitated by the fact that it is now becoming more usual for researchers to make the epistemological orientations and assumptions guiding theory construction and empirical analysis more transparent. In this way, the starting point and the construction principles of theories and methods are made known to other groups of researchers, they become repeatable, and can be critically reviewed. This enables both an appraisal of theoretical and methodological approaches within the overall research design of an epistemological strategy, and a better identification of the relations and overlaps between different theories and methodological approaches.

In recent theory construction, ecological, systemic, and contextualistic paradigms have proved particularly efficient in integrating different scientific theories, and have gained considerable ground both in the three disciplines mentioned (medicine, psychology, and sociology), and in important interdisciplinary research areas such as social medicine, social psychology, social pediatrics, social pedagogy, social epidemiology, and medical psychology:

1. Ecological and systemic models locate the impulses of human development in the reciprocal adaptation and "interpenetration" of organism, individual, and

environment, together forming an organic, psychological, and social system. These systems mutually affect each other, and in the course of development reach a more or less stable equilibrium. Only a stable balance enables an optimal unfolding of personal needs and actions in every dimension: an instable state, however, is the starting point for disorders and diseases.

2. The contextualistic approaches stress the interdependency of human development, on the one hand, and the development of the social and physical environment, on the other: The human subject undergoes a productive process of assimilation and interaction with his or her body and the environment. Specific means are selected to realize specific goals, the consequences of actions are considered, and the fact anticipated that these may change the contextual conditions for the subject's own action. The criterion of a "healthy" development is seen in the acquisition of social, psychological, and physical competencies which enable individuals to act adequately and develop an identity of their own, at the same time taking into account their needs and personality structures.

The theoretical foundations of these approaches have been developed, among others, by Engel (1962), Levi (1975), Lerner (1976), Bronfenbrenner (1979), Magnusson and Allen (1983), and Matarazzo and his associates (1984).

In the following sections, medical, psychological, and sociological models are presented which are inspired by overarching conceptions of the type discussed above, and may therefore play an important role in future interdisciplinary research. Following the review of various theoretical approaches, I will try to outline a comprehensive model for the integration of important parts of these theories in a socialization-theoretical conception.

Medical Approaches

Traditional medical approaches more or less follow a monocausal way of explaining diseases. The early risk-factor model primarily concentrated on relating to a specific single factor releasing a specific result defined in terms of a deficiency, leading to an illness. With the growing importance of chronic illnesses, however, it became obvious that the presence of a single risk factor only allows for a statement of probability and that the interim steps that link the risk factor with the result have to be considered. Thus, traditional linear thinking had to be abandoned, because it does not include feedback effects and multicausal interdependencies.

Recent medical approaches have attempted to compensate for these deficiencies by introducing systemic and contextualistic models. The focussing on purely organic functions has proved insufficient or wholly inapt to explain the origin and development of the recent chronic diseases, thus clearly exposing the limitations of the model of disease of traditional medicine, which is founded on the biochemistry of the human body. Many empirical findings and clinical observations can no longer be accounted for by the traditional model of medicine (Levi 1975):

1. Some individuals react to environmental factors (noxious agents, pathogens, stressors), but others do not.
2. The same type of risk factors or stressors may lead to different illnesses in different individuals.
3. Different types of risk factors or stressor may result in the same illnesses.
4. Some individuals show a disposition toward contracting a particular disease more easily or more frequently than do others.

The linear causal model that has become successfully established in virology can no longer explain these phenomena. Psychological and social variables obviously have to be taken into consideration for their effect on the healthy physiological functioning of the human organism.

Additionally, feedback effects have to be taken into consideration: for example, if an individual loses his or her equilibrium due to physical illness, this may have negative repercussions on other levels. The individual so affected learns something in terms of completely new social experiences, and, in turn, translates them into action. He or she perceives the illness as a psychological threat, becomes a burden on his or her family, has to relinquish certain roles, temporarily or for longer terms, and avails him- or herself of a medical care system designed to provide assistance in coping with the illness. These stresses, and coping with them, in turn affect the biophysical organism, either in a curative capacity or by reinforcing the illness (Petermann, Noecker, & Bode 1987, p. 27). In an analogous form, a social deviance or a psychological disorder may be the starting point for this process (Kessler, Price, & Wortman 1985).

Recent medical approaches envisage a comprehensive model of health and disease, combining the biological, psychological, and sociological aspects of the human organism:

1. Health and disease are considered multifactorally dependent; the predisposition, onset and course of a disease follow certain social, psychological, and physiological rules.
2. Disease is viewed as a failure of adaptation on several levels, not only resulting from damage to the body through a chronic noxious agent or a pathogen, but from maladaption of the organism — as part of the personality in a social context — to stressful situations.
3. Health is defined in terms of a high degree of adaptability of the individual to physical, psychological, and social stressors.

Starting from theoretical premises of this kind, several authors in medical research have attempted to integrate psychological and social factors into a comprehensive model designed to define health and disease. A very interesting example is the model that Kagan and Levi (1985) have developed. In this model, stressful psychosocial stimuli have a key role in acting as risk factors of physiological adaptation and maladaptation. These stimuli are considered potentially health-damaging, at least if they meet with a particular "psychobiological program," which the authors define in terms of a certain disposition and characteristic way in which an individual reacts habitually to environmental demands and social events. This psychobiological program is codetermined by past experiences gained from interacting with the environment, on the one hand, and by genetic factors, on the other.

According to this model, psychosocial stimuli that meet with a specific psychobiological disposition may trigger stress reactions as "mechanisms" for coping. These mechanisms are primarily associated with the physiological reaction of the organism that is elicited by psychosocial stimuli. When the reaction reaches a certain level of intensity, frequency, and duration, in conjunction with specific interacting variables, it may detrimentally affect health or cause illness.

The following concepts are part of this model (Kagan and Levi 1975, p.241):

1. Psychosocial stimuli: They originate in social relations or constellations (i.e., in the environment), influence the organism via processes of the central nervous system, and may cause illness in certain individuals under certain circumstances.
2. Psychobiological program: This describes the tendency to react in accordance with a particular pattern, e.g., in solving a problem or adapting to environmental conditions. The organismic determinants of this program are genetic factors and earlier environmental influences.
3. Mechanisms: These refer to physiological reactions in the organism produced by psychosocial stimuli, which may precipitate the early stages of an illness and cause it to proceed, depending on the intensity, frequency, or duration, and the presence or absence of certain interacting variables. Stress is considered to be a specific mechanism. The term "stress" is used here according to Selye (1956) in order to describe unspecific reactions of the body to certain tasks, a stereotype pattern of adaptation that primes the organism mainly for physical activity, e.g., fighting or fleeing. If physical activity is not possible, or socially undesirable, physical or mental stress may result. Stress is seen as one of the mechanisms that cause illness.
4. Precursors of disease: These refer to functional disorders in psychological or physical systems that may deleteriously affect performance in the long run.
5. Disease: Disease means a reduction in performance due to psychological or somatic malfunctions. A lowering of an individual's performance level indicates failure to cope with certain tasks. In using this definition, it is necessary to specify the biological level of hierarchy that the former refers to. Illness is manifested differently on the cellular, organic, and organismic levels.
6. Interacting variables: They comprise internal or external psychological or somatic factors that alter the effect of causative factors in relation to mechanisms, precursors of disease, or disease itself, i.e., precipitating or slowing down the process resulting in illness.

Figure 1 places these concepts in an overall contextual framework.

The schematic presentation in Fig. 1 makes clear that the psychosocial stimuli, in conjunction with psychobiological programs, are viewed as releasers of emo-

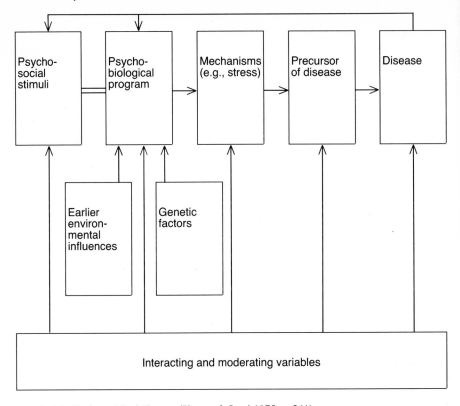

Fig. 1. Medical model of disease (Kagan & Levi 1975, p.241)

tional or biological reactions and responses, and may under certain conditions become precursors of illness. This process is accelerated or slowed down by the interacting variables. It is further assumed that this course of events does not proceed in a linear fashion, but should be visualized as a feedback loop in a cybernetic sense. The authors point out that this model primarily addresses disorders or illnesses of the psychosomatic and chronic types, rather than the traditionally known infectious diseases (see also Matarazzo, Weiss, Herd, Miller, & Weiss 1984; Cohen & Syme 1985).

Complex Psychosomatic and Sociosomatic Models

Other ecological and contextualistic approaches are known as "psychosomatic" or "sociosomatic." In psychosomatic research, the subjective perception of illnesses plays a preeminent role. Somatic complaints are taken to provide information on actual subjective well-being, and on underlying conflicts and their subjective context of meaning. Usually research focusses on such illnesses, in which the psyche of the patient decisively contributes to concrete organic changes and their origin and treatment as well as on somatic complaints without an organic substrate, rooted in psychological conflicts, tensions, and emotions, which may cause a "somatization" or somatic reactions. This research ranks psychological factors both as a cause and a concomitant of illness. Psychosomatics, therefore, rejects a monocausal interpretation of disease and tends to emphasize a subjective context of meaning for the entire course of an illness. Significantly, psychosomatic explanations focus on those illnesses where traditional medicine fails, i.e., chronic diseases or disorders without a pathological background.

The underlying concept of health and disease has been developed by Engel (1962) and recently amplified by the German researchers von Uexküll (1981) and Bräutigam and Christian (1986). According to these authors, disease cannot be sufficiently understood while the reactions of the organism are still being analyzed independently of an individual's social and ecological environment. The predominant view of research has been to study the individual and the environment separately, without a conceptualization of their interrelatedness. As Engel and von Uexküll point out, we can only juxtapose the separate findings obtained by physiological, psychological, or sociological methods. But in order to account for a sick individual in terms of a somato-psycho-social phenomenon, we require models that will help us to interpret the linkages between these three areas.

These authors view illness generally as a failure of adaptive mechanisms — with the subsequent specific diseases representing only certain forms of this failure, but possibly pointing to the same basic psychosocial process. Since physical-noxious agents, viruses, bacteria, psychological conflicts, or social strains produce the same external states, the releasing factor must be something common to all the different, specific causes of illness, which can only be defined as an unspecific noxious agent or detrimental factor. Specific diseases, such as measles, scarlet fever, hypertension, gastric ulcers, depression, etc., would then be no more than variants or different forms of that general state of ill health, and the specific causes of a physical-chemical, biological, psychological, or social kind would be nothing else but variations of a general detrimental effect characteristic of all of them (von Uexküll 1981, p.91).

Of crucial importance in this approach is the degree of actual adaptation to the environment, i.e., the process whereby relations between the individual and the environment develop and change. This is a dynamic process of lifelong, mutual adaptation between the individual and his or her environment, in which even the mature individual has constantly to make adjustments. Seen in this perspective, to be healthy would mean perpetual construction and reconstruction of the concrete relations between the individual and his/her environment, thus enabling a fulfillment of vital needs.

Generally, to be healthy is viewed in terms of a productive shaping and reshaping of the environment; by contrast, to be ill, generally speaking, denotes an ineffective production of environment, followed, after alarm signals, either by adaptation and an overcoming of illness, or — after exhausting available adaptive resources — by disorder or disease. The intricate linkage between somatic, psychological, and social factors is thus conceived of as an integration of programs of varying degrees of complexity for the production of relations between the individual and his/her environment.

The actual starting point for the cause and development of an illness is an overtaxing of the social, psychological, and somatic adaptive potentials of the individual as a bio-psycho-social "system." Both acute and chronic diseases, in particular, place high demands on the regulating capacity of the organism. Excessive strains that initially manifest themselves on the physical level, may over time also affect the psychological and social behavior of a sick individual and vice versa. According to this view, declining health reflects the organism's inability to address particular internal or external organic requirements and cope with them. As with social and psychological normality, so, too, should physical normality be regarded as a state of the individual defined according to specific criteria (Engel 1962).

What is true of social and psychological disorders, to a considerable degree also applies to physical disorders: In every historical period and societal setting, they are subjected to different criteria. There are no universally accepted conceptual tools to describe and analyze the starting point and subsequent development of normal and abnormal physiological states, nor are there any precise criteria for defining the boundary between them. Consequently, the above-mentioned medical conceptions do not visualize health and disease as dichotomous states but in terms of forming a dynamic, reciprocal relationship with fluid transitions. Especially during the early stage of an illness, the "salutogenic" and "pathogenic" mechanisms are in a complex state of balance. If, through supportive measures, the salutogenic processes prevail, they enable an optimal adaptation of the organism; but if the pathogenic processes dominate, a maladaptation occurs, i.e., an inadequate response in terms of what is required. The reciprocity of salutogenesis and pathogenesis is influenced by environmental factors, genetic disposition, life-events, and the psychological motivations of an individual (Garmezy & Rutter 1983; Cohen & Syme 1985; Kessler, Price, & Wortman 1985).

Such a continuum model of health and disease presupposes that through functionally and structurally conditioned states any organism may develop a disposition for stressors to become effective due to internal and external strain, and illness may result. The continuum model also permits us to assume that health can be promoted by increasing the resistance and resilience of the human organism and the personality. The greater an individual's ability to maintain a state of equilibrium in spite of stress, the healthier he or she is. From this point of view, health denotes the strength to live with disorders affecting equilibrium, or reduce and keep them at a certain tolerable level (Kobasa 1979; Boyce 1985). On the other hand, health is also an individual's ability to cope with existing disorders in such a way that self-realization is still possible (Wenzel 1986).

Salutogenic Models

Taking up these considerations, Antonovsky (1979, 1987) has constructed a "salutogenic model" (derived from the Latin salus for health). Rather than asking about the origins of malfunction, his approach is crucially concerned with the question of how individuals manage to stay well and not to show symptoms of disorder or disease. Putting it in one sentence, he is concerned with the question of how it is, in view of the multitude of biologically, psychologically, and socially stressful factors, that individuals still manage to cope with life in the microbiological, biochemical, physical, intrapsychic, social, and cultural spheres of their development.

Antonovsky believes health to be a dynamic interaction between numerous stressful and stress-relieving, protective, and supportive factors. The level of health is the result of a given, but at the same time changeable and vulnerable balance of the relation between potentially harmful and protective factors, that are both internal and external to the individual, have their own history, and may therefore vary in stability. Health or disease are the outcome of an interaction with stressors, in which the context as well as the biography of the individual play a role. The location of an individual on the "ease-disease continuum" is the result of this interaction.

The problem with the traditional definition of "disease" is that it says little about the subjective interpretation by an individual of his or her state. Furthermore, statistics of disease suggest that there exists a nice demarcation between health and disease, when, in fact, there does not. Health and disease, normality and deviation, are all located along one continuum with several dimensions. The individual's position on each of these dimensions is required to decide whether an individual is located nearer the one pole of the ease-disease continuum or the other (Antonovsky 1979).

In all societies, all individuals are exposed throughout their life span to a multitude of stressful factors. The resources available to resist these factors are crucial, in Antonovsky's view, in deciding whether they manifest themselves in more or less strong symptoms of a declining well-being. The resistance potential represents the individual's capacity to cope with given social and biological stressors for that individual's benefit and further development.

Among the resources to resist illness, Antonovsky counts physical, biochemical, material, cognitive, emotional, attitudinal, social, and macrostructural factors, having the effect that pathogenic stressors are either prevented altogether or successfully coped with:

1. In the physical and biochemical field, such resources would be the biologically relevant potentials of the body, rendering it immune against pathogens.
2. In the material field, the reference is to the individual's financial possibilities because money can buy physical safety, protection, and adequate nourishment, i.e., important resources for physical and psychological well-being.

3. As far as the cognitive and emotional powers of resistance are concerned, the main factor is intelligence in the sense of flexibility and rationality in adapting to environmental conditions.
4. The interpersonal social resources focus on the social support of different dimensions that an individual's network holds in store.
5. The macrostructural resistance potential refers primarily to the degree of cultural integration of a society: If a system of orientation is available that offers to every individual a position within the social structure, and conveys to him or her a sense of being respected, and of the meaningfulness of his or her own actions, this is an optimal starting point for salutary behavior.

According to Antonovsky's theory, the resources of resistance (i.e., coping) are especially effective in counteracting stressors when the previous biography of a person has been positive and marked by a strong "sense of coherence." Antonovsky uses this term (1979, p.123) to describe the global orientation of an individual that refers to the measure of a generalized, enduring, and dynamic sense of confidence on the part of the individual that his or her own internal and external environment is predictable, coupled with the possibility that things will develop as one would reasonably expect them to. Thus, the "sense of coherence" concept defines a positive self-image in relation to action competence, to the manageability of the internal and external conditions of life and to the individual's belief in being able to control and shape his or her life, thus deriving a subjective meaningfulness and reconciling it with subjective desires and needs. The sense of coherence expresses the extent to which a person has a feeling of confidence that the personal and social resources are available to him/her or meet the demands posed by the stimuli from the environment and that these demands are challenges worthy of investment and engagement (Antonovsky 1987, p.19).

Figure 2 presents a simplified version of Antonovsky's salutogenic model. It demonstrates the degree of complexity that Antonovsky envisages for the interplay between the various moderating factors (general resistance resources, types of life experiences, sense of coherence, successful/unsuccessful tension management) operating between the two poles of the "stressors" and the "health-disease continuum."

On a critical note, one could say that the very complexity of the model — which is only partially conveyed by Fig. 2 — is also its weakness. Furthermore, the attempt to account for all conceivable stressors and for all conceivable resistance resources, from the genetic to the macrosocietal, in a single model, appears not wholly practicable at the present time. Clearly though, Antonovsky's model constitutes a stimulating, thought-provoking contribution to interdisciplinary theory and research. The model raises questions about health that are to be addressed by all the scientific disciplines mentioned here, and therefore presents a considerable integrative potential.

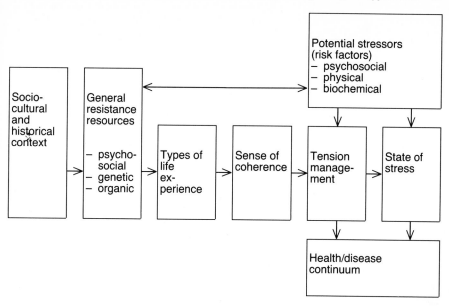

Fig. 2. The salutogenic model, simplified version (Antonovsky 1979, pp.184–185)

Psychological Approaches

In psychological research, too, there have been increased efforts recently to develop multifactorial and multicausal explanatory models that include psychological, physical, and social factors. From the perspective of developmental psychology, it has to be clarified to what extent health-endangering or health-promoting conditions are identical to development-endangering or development-promoting circumstances. Depending on the viewpoint and the concrete questions asked, human development is regarded as a condition or an outcome of health; which developmental characteristics are an important or even sufficient precondition of health depends on the criteria applied to determine and evaluate health and development (Ulich 1987, p.164).

Modern research into developmental psychology is considerably influenced by the stress-coping paradigm. It envisages a high probability for the occurrence of disorders and disease, whenever stress-enforcing factors outweigh the factors protecting against stress. A diminishing of protective factors, e.g., owing to change in, or loss of, social and material support, a decline of the individual's power of resistance, negative changes in the life situation, loss of skills and competencies and of physical energy, can increase the likelihood of a psychological or physiological disorder whenever heavy demands are being made on an individual's coping ability.

Developmental Models

Research in developmental psychology mainly focusses on the identification of personal coping and stress-management styles, devoting particular attention to those features that dispose an individual toward reacting unduly to physical, psychological, and social stressors. These persons have a low degree of resilience; they are "vulnerable." Vulnerability denotes a personal disposition that reacts with exaggerated sensitivity to any kind of change in well-being because the set of personal abilities available for the processing of reality are relatively unstable and low on self-confidence. Vulnerable individuals, much more than less vulnerable ones, tend to report more — and more vividly — on critical life-events and everyday stresses: They show a comparatively high perceptiveness to stressors within their social life setting (Murphy & Moriarty 1976).

Rather than being concerned only with clarifying the impact of personal attributes that lead to vulnerability or resistance to stressors, further developments of this theoretical approach increasingly try to bring in social aspects and resources in addition to the personal (psychological and physical) ones, since the reciprocal effect and reinforcement of the factors involved is obvious (Garmezy & Rutter 1983).

A convincing conception, supported by elaborate empirical longitudinal studies, has been presented by Werner and Smith (1982). Their work rests on a survey of a cohort of children born in 1955 that was conducted over a period of more than 20 years. Parents and teachers were also included in the study. During the initial phase of the study, 72 out of 695 children were selected because they showed an accumulation of serious risk factors, such as poor family background, perinatally sustained impairments, genetic defects, and a sick mother, but who show up no marked symptoms of any psychological disorders during the first years of life. In spite of their specific physical, psychological, and social disadvantages, they developed "powers of resistance" to the unfavorable conditions of their lives, which in turn protected them against psychological disorders.

The study by Werner and Smith demonstrably shows that some of the children did not manifest disorders during their subsequent life course, as might have been expected, but proceeded to develop in good mental and social health, despite the following grave risk factors:

1. Persistent poverty
2. Considerable complications during birth
3. Noticeable retardations and disorders affecting development
4. Psychopathological illness of parents
5. Genetic abnormalities and hereditary defects
6. Low educational level of mother

They had become psychologically "resilient," because they were able, for instance, to cope effectively with stressful situations in an active and productive manner, and establish positive relations of a compensatory nature with other individuals, thereby initiating for themselves positive feedback on their coping capacity.

The authors distinguish between stressful and supportive factors in the socializational environment of a child. These could also be called detective and protective factors, which can reinforce or diminish the impact of risk factors and the resultant increased vulnerability toward deviance, disorders, and impairments. Some of the stressful environmental factors were identified as follows:

1. Longer periods of separation from the primary caregiver during the first year of life
2. Birth of sibling(s) during the first two years of life
3. Serious or repeated childhood diseases
4. Siblings with disabilities or problem behavior
5. Enduring disharmony in the family
6. Absence of father
7. Unemployment of parents
8. Move of the family
9. Change of school
10. Divorce of parents
11. Arrival of a step-parent in the home
12. Departure or death of an older sibling

Protective factors were found to be the following:

1. At least two years age difference between siblings
2. High measure of attention given to the child during first year of life
3. Positive parent-child relationship during first years of life
4. Presence of reference individuals in addition to mother
5. Receiving good care from siblings and grandparents
6. Availability of relatives and neighbors for emotional support
7. Clear-cut structures and norms in the home
8. Close peer relations
9. Good opportunities for obtaining advice from kindergarten teachers, school teachers, priests, etc.
10. Good access to specialized services, such as health authorities, counseling agencies, etc.
11. Contentedness of mother due to permanent employment
12. Values and life perspectives shared by all family members

The study demonstrates that only by simultaneously accounting, at the same time, for the stressful and the supportive factors present in the socializational environment of a child can the course of development be reconstructed, that is, proceeding from risk factors to either "normal" or "abnormal" forms of behavior. According to the study, resilience and vulnerability factors are reciprocal in their effect and — in combination with other personality traits, specific coping and stress management styles as well as an individual's temperament and character — operate as a filter that reinforces, neutralizes, or diminishes risk factors.

The presence of the "vulnerability" factor during personality development due to the existence of risk factors does not lead directly and inevitably to symptoms

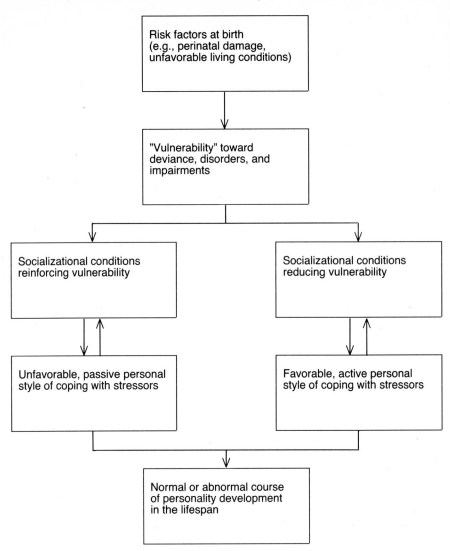

Fig. 3. Interrelatedness of risk factors and courses of development (Werner & Smith 1982)

of deviance, disorder, and impairment, but is moderated in its impact by favorable, individual coping styles and social resources. Figure 3 gives a schematic illustration of this.

Models of Person-Environment Fit

Explanatory approaches of this developmental kind provide a good orientation for theory construction also in neighboring fields of psychological research. In particular, I would like to mention the "fitting" model, based on behavior or action theory. According to this model, the individual interacts more or less appropriately with his or her inner and outer nature in trying to fulfill inner and outer requirements. Considerable deficits in the "fit" between the individual's own abilities and aspirations and the physiopsychological as well as environmental demands placed on him or her, may cause behavior disorders in the areas of social action, thought and imagination, emotions, and organic functions. Overburdening or strain, accompanied by a considerable decline in physical, psychological, and social "well-being," may occur as a result of such an interaction with inner and outer demands, which may impede further development in terms of individuation and social integration (Kaplan 1983).

The emphasis of this explanatory approach is on the process underlying the origin and development of disorders. Behavior is seen as a symptom of and/or reaction to overtaxing and excessive demands confronting the adaptive mechanisms, e.g., when children and adolescents are not able to meet the demands made on them within and outside the family and by other educational institutions, or when adults are not able to meet the demands of partnership or professional life.

Such an overload interferes with performance, e.g., producing lack of concentration and motivation for learning or leads to problem behavior, such as difficulties in establishing interpersonal relations, aggressiveness, emotional disorders, feelings of inadequacy, psychosomatic disorders, etc. This overtaxing of a person's coping potentials in turn affects the social environment and elicits additional stressors, involving parents, colleagues, or peers in problem-laden conflicts, and demanding of them specific adaptive achievements (Pearlin & Lieberman 1979; Farran & McKinney 1986).

According to this theoretical approach, a person interacts with his or her environment, but cannot cope with the inner and outer tasks involved in the process. Maladaptations, which are not just of a temporary nature but are part of any normal developmental process, lead to internal and external conflicts. Frequent and persistent maladaptations cause serious deficits in the fit between an individual's own abilities and the demands posed by the environment. Problem behavior is therefore primarily regarded as an individual's attempt to solve the problems he or she has with his or her own body and the environment (Coleman 1980; Brim & Kagan 1980).

From the mismatch between situational tasks and the individual's own behavior options, he or she develops coping strategies that are regarded by the social environment as pathogenic or deviant. To this extent, behavior disorders are also indicators of deficient or inadequate competencies and skills. These deficiencies have to be seen in the context of an individual's previous learning and experiential opportunities and life setting, since the latter reflect on the individual's own history of coping with the demands posed by the social environment.

A behavior disorder may therefore be interpreted as an instance of problem solving that is not acceptable to the reference groups. The judgment and the normative decisions of reference persons and groups are constitutive for the development of the disorder, and may both initiate and reinforce it. Problem behavior is not seen as an objective fact indwelling in the individual, but as a response that sometimes turns into deviance only because it is measured against the social norms and judgments of a reference group (Jessor & Jessor 1977; Silbereisen, Eyferth, & Rudinger 1986).

The person-environment approach to explaining deviance and disorder stimulates further research into the mechanisms that mediate and convey biophysical and psychosoical dimensions of human development and lead to a healthy personality (Baltes, Featherman, & Lerner 1986). Future investigations should direct attention to the social resources of support, especially the structural anchoring and the course of interaction in socializational agencies and other informal and formal institutions. Explanations of "unsuccessful" interaction with the social environment and the individual's own psychosocial development have to be sought in the context of conditions and structures of interaction in the family, at school, with the peer group, at the workplace, etc., all of which are themselves part of the socioeconomic and ecological environmental constellation (Lerner 1982).

Sociological Approaches

Modern sociological approaches have included several of the theoretical premises that have already been discussed in connection with the medical and psychological conceptions. In comparison, sociological approaches give more emphasis to the economic, ecological, and cultural influences on human behavior which is relevant for health. Recently, the long neglected importance of physical and psychological characteristics and dispositions has been increasingly acknowledged.

Recent approaches have overcome the limited, functionalist conception that had been developed from the theoretical position of Parsons (1951). Parsons was one of the first sociologists who systematically addressed the role of health and disease in modern industrialized societies. In his approach, the principal prerequisite for the development of societal well-being in industrialized societies is the absence of any interference with the normal functioning of the organism. Its undisturbed functioning is the basis not only of physical, but also of social and occupational efficiency (Parsons 1951a, p.75).

Parson's point of departure, therefore, is the high demand confronting every adult individual in respect to his/her contribution to the functioning of the social system. He argues that the social value of an individual in contemporary societies is determined in terms of achievements that are judged by others. The more freely available and applicable the human achievement potential, the more an individual is of value to society. Sociologically defined, somatic health is the state of optimal ability to effectively fulfill tasks deemed valuable. Health can be defined as the state of an individual's optimal efficiency in fulfilling the tasks for which he or she has been socialized. It is thus defined in relation to the individual's share in the social system. Accordingly, disease would be categorically defined as a generalized interference affecting an individual's potential to fulfill tasks normally expected of him or her (Parsons 1951a, p.71).

Parsons's conception thus rests on a highly mechanistic view of the connection between societal demands and individual behavior. Within the context of his approach, he allows for the possibility of a retreat into illness as being a response to role overload (Parsons 1951b). For Parsons, the problem of health is tied up with the utilization, typical of capitalist industrial societies, by work organizations of a fully efficient body, i.e., a human being is perceived merely as a unit of potential performance (cf. Navarro 1976).

The problem with this conception is that it does not address the dynamics operating between social demands, psychological strain, and physical symptoms of illness; the underlying assumption is that of an isolated concept of the human organism being a vegetatively controlled system. Although Parsons discusses the interrelatedness of social demands and physical disorders in his comprehensive theoretical design, and has thus contributed valuable perspectives to subsequent sociological research, the moderating significance of the psychological system (personality), which is an element of his theoretical conception, has not been fully accounted for.

Social Lifestyle Models

Recent sociological and social epidemiological models, similar to the models discussed earlier, take into account psychosocial risk factors associated with environmental conditions that may cause serious, sometimes enduring strains, resulting in considerable maladaptation of the physical, psychological, and social capacities. These approaches share the assumption that psychosocial risks arise from the discrepancy between human needs, abilities, and expectations, on the one hand, and the given possibilities for fulfilling particular behavioral tasks, on the other. As "moderating factors," both social factors (mediated by the existing value system and the social structure), on the one hand, and personal factors (mediated by genetic conditions), on the other, are included.

These "intervening variables" produce effects that are more or less psychosocially protective and have a neutralizing or exacerbating influence on stressors. Taken together, social support and coping styles constitute a "psychosocial immune system" insofar as they fulfill a protective or supportive function in the resistance to psychosocial risks and their outcomes. For a number of chronic diseases and their genesis, such as hypertension, heart conditions, bronchial asthma, gastric and intestinal ulcers, and circulatory disorders, evidence in support of this model has been gathered in numerous empirical studies (Strauss 1975; Wiley & Camacho 1980; House 1981a; Badura 1983; Berkman & Breslow 1983; Mechanic 1982; Clausen 1984; Kessler & McLeod 1985).

In some of these approaches, the concept of lifestyle serves a general organizing function. It denotes the patterns and structures of behaviors that occur as a result of coping with daily routines, persistent strains, or critical life-cycle transitions. The term "lifestyle" refers to the more or less culturally accepted individual and collective behavior strategies that have evolved in response to such events and that serve to control and manage the resultant problems of adaptation (Sobel 1982). If these habitual strategies become stabilized in an unproductive manner, we can speak of health-endangering and risk-carrying lifestyles. Examples are alcohol consumption, smoking, wrong diet, and lack of physical exercise (Wiley & Camacho 1980). Such health-endangering lifestyles may arise in connection with certain social, economic, cultural, and political conditions. In industrial societies, they seem to have reached epidemic proportions.

Typically, in today's social environment, numerous stimuli and informal pressures exist that contribute to a health-endangering lifestyle (Badura 1983, p.40). The concept of lifestyle embraces the relatively stable set of health-relevant action patterns that develops in the course of biographical processes and within concrete social relationships. These habitual patterns need not necessarily be consciously available to the individual. Lifestyle reflects specific patterns of problem solving and coping that are related to a particular social context. In this sense, lifestyle is the sum of patterns of meaning and forms of expression that are the outcome of the collective efforts undertaken by human beings to cope with the demands and contradictions inherent in social structures and settings (Wenzel 1986).

Only by relating the concept of lifestyle really closely to sociostructural conditions can its critical potential be fully exploited. We should not restrict the concept of lifestyle to consumption-oriented manifestations of behavior, as is sometimes done in social psychology. Rather, the reference here is to a behavior-relevant inquiry into the entire ecology of the societal living conditions. In addition to family life and leisure, these primarily include the conditions of work, i.e., the exploitation of human labor in work organizations. As has been pointed out, in today's Western societies it is structurally difficult for the individual and for specific groups to coordinate and synthesize the various demands stemming from the different areas and fields of everyday life. Thus, the lifestyle approach tries to encompass the totality of an individual's or a group's range of activities as determined by economic, social, and natural-ecological living conditions, including the production of material and intellectual goods in the political and domestic spheres, as well as leisure activities and intimate social contacts (Smelser & Erikson 1980).

Sociological Stress Theories

As with the medical and psychological concepts, sociological research, too, has developed stress-theoretical models addressing the connection between various stressors and behavior outcomes and including personal and social moderating variables. A well-structured model has been presented by Leonard I. Pearlin. He has attempted to integrate the various medical and psychological approaches to the concept of stress into a sociological concept. To Pearlin, the concept of stress, despite its broad definition, is useful in sociological terms, because it calls attention to the individual's interaction with the social environment. In his view, the stress concept serves both an inner psychological analysis of personal reactions and a linking up of these with the surrounding social conditions. It enables a theoretical linkage between the social and inner emotional lives of individuals (Pearlin 1987).

Pearlin's explanatory model starts from social and economic conditions, that is, age, sex, social class, occupational status, race or ethnic group, and other ascribed characteristics as well as institutionalized role context (family, school, workplace, neighborhood, etc.), all of which elicit stressors and strains and thus lead to manifestations of stress symptoms. In addition, he includes social mediators (especially activities in the political sphere insofar as they relate to the social framework conditions and collective actions initiated by the individuals affected) and personal mediators, including coping capacities (see Fig. 4).

The stressors in this model are those conditions that cause an individual to perceive instances of insecurity, threat, or strain, and may therefore act as triggers for stress symptoms. The definition of stressors is kept deliberately wide-ranging, and comprises an extensive spectrum of potential triggers. Pearlin distinguishes the following categories of psychosocial risks:

1. Critical life-events, for example, unexpected loss of an important reference person, separation or divorce, sudden onset of a serious illness, change of workplace
2. Chronic tensions, for example, role conflicts and role ambiguities owing to the twofold burden of work and household duties, physical and nervous stress at the workplace, persistent work overload, unfulfilled career expectations, enduring conflicts with a partner/spouse, emotional conflicts with children, long-term illnesses
3. Difficult transitions in the life cycle, for example, from childhood to adulthood, from school to employment, from employment to retirement

This categorization tempers the significance of critical life-events. Rather than emphasizing the stressful impact of the cumulation of several different, critical life-events, Pearlin focusses on the radiating effect of each of the individual events for the social integration into the social network, the mobilization of coping competencies, self-image, and psychological and physical well-being. From a sociological perspective, many problems confronting individuals during their lives are not of an extraordinary nature but instead pose enduring problems that have to be overcome by each individual while playing his or her everyday social role in the societal institutions such as the working sphere or the family or in respect to the person's capacity as a superior, employee, spouse, or housewife (Pearlin & Lieberman 1979).

The chronic stress associated with the work environment, for example, has so far received little attention, although, according to the findings of Pearlin, it may in the long run affect the individual's state of health considerably. The impact of

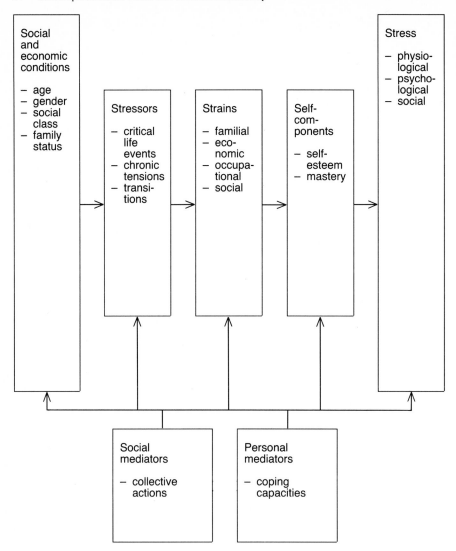

Fig. 4. A sociological model of the stress-strain process (Pearlin 1987, p.60)

such stress has been underestimated because research has primarily concentrated on the psychological and physical implications of acute job insecurity, of pressure on the individual to increase performance, of physically or chemically dangerous working conditions, etc., and has tended to neglect such longer-term stressors as an unfavorable work environment, monotonous or fragmented work, few opportunities for contacts with colleagues, limited scope for action and career prospects, conflict-laden working relations with superiors, colleagues, and inferiors. It is obvious, though, that these enduring stresses contribute to the development of lifestyles that endanger and damage health, leading to consumption of alcohol and nicotine, psychological ailments, and physical disorders (Kasl 1979).

Pearlin attaches much weight to continuous physical, psychological, and role-based stressors of everyday life, especially where they affect central elements of an individual's everyday behavior. Persistent conflicts and subsequent tensions as well as frustrated expectations in relation to marital and other relationships, parent-child relations, or the workplace, may — sometimes in connection with the sudden occurrence of a trivial event, and sometimes for no apparent reason at all — trigger psychological and physical stress symptoms. It is the persistent, recurring strain on the individual's self-esteem rather than the unexpected event itself that provides the background to disorders and diseases (Pearlin 1983).

According to Pearlin, continuing stress due to conflicts and acute stressful events are interrelated. For example, critical life-events may be stressful for the simple reason that they exacerbate an already existing role strain, or mark the beginning of long-term role strain, for example, when, owing to the death of a spouse, there is an overburdening from parental duties and employment, or when sudden unemployment leads to tensions in partner relations and affects the financial circumstances of the family (Pearlin 1987, p.56).

The personal and social mediating factors influence processes leading to the manifestation of stress, and eventually determine whether or not a stressor leads to an overtaxing of the adaptive capacities and coping abilities of an individual. Pearlin points out that all stressors may be part of the institutional arrangements and social structures of society, and for this reason at least some of these can only be influenced by public policies or collective actions. The social context that provides the starting point of any process leading to stress symptoms cannot be altered by way of individual coping strategies, but only through collective actions and political measures.

If this fact is overlooked, the attempt to strengthen individual coping capacities will only end in further demoralization and experiences of failure of the individual concerned. The significance of individual coping abilities is thus not denied, but put in perspective. In Pearlin's view, the personal mediating factors are crucial in raising self-esteem and a sense of personal efficiency, controllability, and self-reliance. Again, a lowering of self-esteem and of the feeling that one is losing control of one's own life ("locus of control") is more likely to happen if long-lasting, chronic role strains and stresses due to living and working conditions are present (Pearlin 1987, p.58).

This model views psychological disorders and physical illnesses as symptoms and manifestations of conflicting social events and processes. Manifestations of stress can be observed at the different levels of the entire personality, both on the level of the organism, that is, the physical functioning of the different organs, the functioning of the endocrine and immunological system, and on the level of psychological, emotional, cognitive, and social behavior; malfunctioning on one level invariably leads to disruptions on another.

A Socialization-Theoretical Synthesis

As the review of different theoretical approaches has shown, there are many connecting lines between the individual models. In order to develop synthesis, I will try to integrate some crucial parts of the theories and models into a socialization-theoretical concept.

Recent theoretical approaches in socialization research are based on the assumption that societal and natural (environmental) factors and biopsychological (personal) factors jointly affect personality development. The relations between the individual and his/her environment are viewed in terms of a complex reciprocity. Socialization describes the lifelong process of personality development as proceeding on a basis of mutual dependence of, and continuous interaction with, the societally mediated, social and material environment, on the one hand, and with the biophysical structure of the organism, on the other. Programmatically, the concept refers to the fact that the human individual, due to changes in the biological and the environmental conditions, is in a permanent state of development (Hurrelmann 1988).

Following this approach, the development of the human personality can be linked to the mutual relationship between the biological organism and the social and material environment. Personality denotes the individual's specific, organized structure of characteristics, qualities, attitudes. skills, and action competencies that has evolved on the basis of the individual's biological constitution, as a biographical result of interacting and coping with the demands posed by life. Human personality development, then, could be described as a sequential and long-term changing of crucial elements of this structure during the life course (Goslin 1969; Wentworth 1980).

A specific example of the individual-environment model is the "model of the productive processing of reality" (Hurrelmann 1988). Personality development is here understood as a largely self-directed process, involving, in a complex manner, conditions of life that are both internal and external to the organism. Personality development is assumed to occur at the interface of a "subjective" and an "objective" factor, of inner and outer reality.

In the model of the productive processing of reality, the individual is viewed as one who interacts with the environment in a searching and sounding-out manner, on the one hand, and who constructively intervenes and is creative, on the other. The individual assimilates environmental factors and reconciles them with existing views and potentials, and, at the same time, endeavors to achieve an equilibrium between environmental demands and his or her own needs, interests, and abilities, both motoric and physical.

The model envisages a social and material environment that is undergoing constant change and reorganization, and is influenced and altered throughout by activities undertaken by individuals. Influence and change in turn affect the process of perceiving, assimilating, processing, coping with, and structuring reality.

At the same time, the concept proposes a certain view of society: A social system created and further developed by human beings. The model of the productive processing of reality reflects the dual character of social systems. As a given fact, they provide an objective framework for living whose validity extends beyond the individual life; individuals become integrated into it, but via subjective acquisition, it is being permanently reconstructed. Through being productively processed, social reality can only be preserved and passed on if it is assimilated by the next generation in a productive way. Essential to this view of society is the idea that in principle it is possible to overcome social constraints and power relations, and to decide freely on the future structuring of one's life.

This concept of socialization seeks to overcome the traditional neglect of genetic and biological dimensions of development which has been typical for relevant theories in sociology (Featherman & Lerner 1985). It is quite obvious that the biogenetic potentials of cellular, muscular, and organic systems affect the skills and abilities of individuals, and determine the basis for behavior — just as any change in the ecological and social environment stimulates adaptive activities on the psychological, physiological, sensory, cognitive, emotional, and social levels. Over the entire life course, we have to take into consideration the interplay between organic, psychological, and social areas of personality development. Biophysical and biochemical processes affect psychological dispositions, and social and ecological factors influence the chronology and microstructures of all developmental processes in all age periods and phases of the life cycle (Soerensen, Weinert, & Sherrod 1986; Clausen 1986b).

A comprehensive socialization-theoretical conception of personality development has to account for the somatic and motoring dimensions as well as the biogenetic disposition. The relationship of the individual to his or her own body can be defined in two ways. On the one hand, it is defined biogenetically — body and movement cannot be controlled arbitrarily and randomly. The human individual as a species is subject to biological limitations. Every individual has a specific, biogenetic potential, and in the course of ontogenesis, a realization of biogenetic programs of development can be expected. On the other hand, the relationship is defined in social terms. Body and movement are social structures because cultural rules, norms, and definitions suggest or prescribe to the individual how to relate to his or her body.

A Synthesis Model

As has been shown, recent medical, psychological, and sociological approaches apply epistemological models of the ecological, systemic, and contextualist type, which are very close to this interdisciplinary conception of socialization theory. Obviously, the concept of socialization, as outlined above, has several commonalities with the medical, psychological, and sociological theories. Therefore, attempting to integrate the main parts of the various theories discussed, using "sozialization" as a frame work concept, proves expedient.

If we draw together the most important elements and variables from the models discussed above, we arrive at the synthesis model shown in Fig. 5.

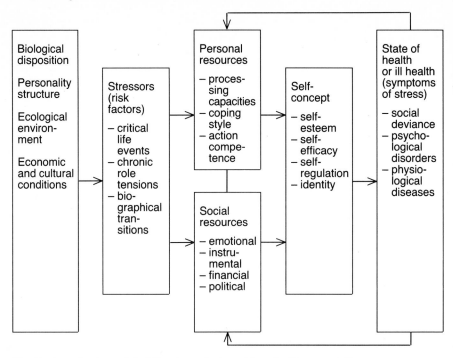

Fig. 5. A synthesis model of the stress-deviance/disorder/disease relation

It is important to note that the synthesis model views deviance, disorder, and disease as being a result of an "unsuccessful" socialization process. It thereby incorporates some of the main concepts of biophysical and salutogenic theories, the stress-coping model, developmental theories, and sociological theories. The crucial starting point for any type of disorder is seen in the inadequacy both of intrapersonal and interpersonal capacities for coping with age- and situation-specific demands for action and behavior. Just as in the various approaches mentioned above, a risk constellation for the origin of disorders is considered present, if and when, due to specific personal and environmental characteristics, only inappropriate and inadequate individual and/or social resources are available to an individual in one or several important spheres of action, so that skills and abilities expected and required by the social environment cannot be exercised.

Whether or not the process of socialization succeeds, depends on the adequacy of individual action competencies and the social support potential available for the various tasks confronting the individual. If the personal as well as the social resources are insufficiently developed in an individual's life setting in terms of structure and profile, the preconditions and foundations needed for self-efficacious and self-regulated behavior will be lacking, and the probability increases that physiologically, psychologically, and socially deviant forms of action and behavior will develop.

In epistemological terms, this approach does not distinguish between the explanations of the development of deviance, disorder, and disease, nor does it distinguish between the explanation of health and ill health, well-being and disease.

To sum up, the following, principal statements of the previously discussed theories on the stress-health-disease relation are part of the socialization-theoretical conception:

1. Whether or not specific constellations of stressful situations, events, and life situations (e.g., strain at school or the workplace, difficulties in establishing interpersonal relations, problematic life-cycle transitions) lead to problem behavior depends first and foremost on the individual's specific skills and abilities to cope with stressors. For example, if a discrepancy is perceived between action competencies and actions to be performed, the individual has to mobilize strategies to overcome the former. These strategies can be developed if and when there is the ability and readiness on the part of the individual to realistically perceive and assess his or her own action competencies and to identify as precisely as possible in which areas a discrepancy exists in relation to the competencies required. Following this diagnosis, strategies that are adequate to the situation have then to be implemented to correct and control individual action competencies, on the one hand, and the situational demands for action, on the other, in order to eliminate the discrepancy.

2. The personal resources available for coping with stressful situations and events are, in part, contingent on the course of personality development and biography. The possibilities and patterns of constructing strategies for coping behavior are influenced, directly and indirectly, by the social and material living conditions. Using a socialization approach, the close connections between these aspects can easily be made transparent, since the interrelatedness of personal individuation and the social integration of the individual is one of the central postulates of this theoretical approach. Apart from individual coping strategies and the personal resources they reflect, the social resources, from a socialization theoretical viewpoint, are an important moderating factor that determine whether or not stress leads to problem behavior. As indicated above, the social resources can be defined in terms of the potential material, financial, informational, instrumental, emotional, cultural, and social stimuli, as well as support by the environment available to the individual in a specific life situation.

3. From a socialization-theoretical standpoint, symptoms of an impairment of the normal social, psychological, and physical development can also be considered as indicators of deficient interactional and communication processes in the context of socialization, that is, within the family, school, peer group, occupational, and leisure organizations, etc. In such a case, the agencies of socialization have not been capable of providing effective impulses and support for reconciling the opportunities and demands for action present in the environment with the action competencies of the individual. In relation to a given situation, the capacities for action are deficient because the support provided by the agencies of socialization has been inadequate.

4. Whether or not the incidence of stressful events, as they occur in everyday life, is coped with and compensated in a way conducive to and promoting further personality development depends on the form of personal and social resources. If favorable resources are available, self-esteem, self-efficacy, self-regulation, and identity can be developed in a balanced way. In the case of unfavorable resources, behavior disorder may ocur in stressful situations because the individual concerned does not respond to the physical, psychological, and social challenges in a manner that is socially accepted and recognized, and that is beneficial to further personality development.

5. Status transitions and new tasks during the life course represent stages at which the demands confronting the individual change quickly and markedly. The development during a transitional period can be effectively coped with if the individual is facing a limited measure of changes and situational challenges. The transition period can then serve a necessary reprogramming and extension of the existing behavior repertoire. A successful fulfillment of demands denotes a constellation that is perceived subjectively and classified as successful. The demands made on behavior seem to the individual to be challenges he or she has to deal with successfully. However, if the demands exceed the existing behavior repertoire and put a strain on the coordination of the various behavior programs in the different areas undergoing development, there is the danger of an unsuccessful coping with the situation. Various types of mechanisms, such as opposition, evasion, withdrawal, conflict, and aggression, are activated in such circumstances and may cause deviance, disorder, or physical illnesses, according to the most "vulnerable" level or system affected.

Every individual has thus to be regarded as a "productive processor of reality," in that he or she realizes an active achievement in coping with tasks and demands typical of a situation, a phase of life, or a particular age: At every turn of the genesis and development of deviance, disorder and disease, a dynamic searching and sounding process is set in motion that leads to a reorganization of personal and social resources and of the self-concept.

Health, Identity, and Lifestyle

The socialization-theoretical model outlined above, which shows a similarity with recent medical and psychological concepts, points to the importance of health-oriented behavior, understood as social behavior learned within a social context and acquired during the life course. The individual's abilities for coping are formed in the course of a lifelong acquisition of and interaction with his or her own body in its ecological and social settings; they are the results as well as the resultants of this process. For this reason, individual coping behavior is intimately related to the interactional and social structures of the person's environment, and thus to the structures of power and inequality of society.

Uta Gerhard (1979) has proposed an analytical distinction between psychophysiological, psychological, and social dimensions of coping behavior in order to identify the different analytical levels of organism, psyche, and social environment:

1. The psychophysiological coping capacities refer to the adjustment of the body to crucial life changes and physical stress.
2. Psychological coping behavior focusses on an effective, subjective structuring of meanings, and the appraisal as well as the making available of ways of psychological processing.
3. The social coping behavior of an individual denotes an active influencing of the environment to improve his or her own position in coping with difficult life-events, situations, and transitions.

The development of active coping strategies presupposes, on the one hand, the ability to employ the social resources effectively. This approach enables a linkage to be established between individual action competencies and social resources for action, which are influenced by the opportunities and power structures of society at large. Individual coping capacity also includes seeking help from external sources, and changing the situational conditions for action to reduce the type and degree of stress.

On the other hand, coping behavior — as a social action in the sense outlined above — presupposes the processing of information derived by way of the individual's perception and observation of his or her own activities during the process of interaction with the social and ecological environment as well as with his/her own body and its needs, all of which contribute towards the establishment of the self-concept. The self-concept mirrors the subjective assessment of the individual's characteristics as well as previous experiences gained in implementing abilities and skills during the interaction with inner and outer reality.

Coping behavior is thus possible only if there is a subjective continuity of the individual's own experience on the basis of his or her self-concept. This continuity of the experience of "being identical with oneself" ("identity") relates both to the various biographical stages and the different social action competencies peculiar to these stages, as well as to the various action fields in which an individual is active (Hurrelmann 1988, p.169).

Identity should always be conceived of as an individual's process of coordination that runs in two directions: Identity is established if and when the interaction with inner and outer reality has yielded solutions that are compatible with each other. As such, the structure of the needs and interests of an individual as well as his or her action competency need not be in complete agreement with the institutionally and organizationally defined social expectations of the environment. Rather, to be able to achieve coordination means to be able to cope with, resolve, or actively deal with tensions that necessarily result from the discrepancy between an individual's own needs, competencies, and social requirements.

The reflexive relationship of an individual to his or her existential living conditions, on the one hand, and the inner structure of his or her own needs, motives and interests, on the other, is a difficult one to establish and maintain under present-day living and working conditions. The increasing process of deinstitutionalization of norms and values, and the diminishing opportunities for sensual experiences in everyday life due to the pervasive influence of the media pose considerable demands on the coordination and control of an individual's action. Separate segments of life that develop by way of differentiation into societal subsystems with specific institutional and organizational features involve a risk of the individual inasmuch as he or she is likely to perceive, assess, and experience him- or herself differently in different spheres of life. The growing compartmentalization of the spheres of life poses increasing risks for a successful formation of identity, as does the pressure for a more individualized structuring of life-cycle transitions, rendering an individual's biography susceptible to unexpected disruptions and readjustments (Meyer 1986).

Establishing and maintaining the continuity of an individual's self-experience is thus precarious at any given moment of his or her life. At the same time, continuity is expected by our societies, and ranks highly among its values (Elias 1987, p.196). Identity is part of a personality structure that exists in the form familiar to us, and is required only in the context of the specific characteristics of our present historical framework; but it also constitutes an expected ideal for every individual living in today's society.

In the formation of an identity, each individual depends on the culturally evolved, collective forms of interaction with society and nature. They are acquired during his or her development and lifetime in an individual, unique fashion, yet they remain within a socially predetermined framework. Political power structures, economic relations of production, patterns of social inequality, hierarchies of cultural norms and values, patterns of processing and manipulation of the physical environment, as well as certain accepted notions of interaction with one's own body — these are the collective parameters circumscribing the scope and opportunities of the individual's forms of expression of self-concept and identity.

The biological, psychological, and sociological dimensions of health and ill health, well-being and disease, can appropriately be subsumed under the concept of lifestyle. As previously mentioned, this concept comprises the physical, psychological, and social components pertaining to individual and collective behavior in a concrete life setting. The lifestyle of a social group refers to the totality of patterns of meaning and forms of expression that evolve in the course of collective efforts made by the group to cope with the demands and inconsistencies inherent in the social structure and the situations affecting its members. The lifestyle reveals what sort of (re-)actions a social group develops under what sort of living conditions, and thus tells us something about the action-guiding orientations a group is capable of developing in the continuous interaction with its living conditions. These orientations, in the form of shared social values, norms, language codes, interaction rituals, etc., constitute a reservoir for individuals or subgroups from which they draw their personal and social identity; it enables them to give meaning and significance to their specific life situation (Erben, Franzkowiak, & Wenzel 1986, p.86).

Individuals develop their personal lifestyles in the course of personality development through the acquisition of, and interaction with, their natural and societal environment. In doing so, each individual refers to the reservoir of values, norms, and action patterns provided by his or her social group and mediated during socialization, but makes use of it in an individualized manner, giving it idiosyncratic emphases (Simmons 1981). Individual lifestyle, which is characterized by certain structures of processing and coping as well as patterns of self-concept is anchored in the social structure and in the cultural and ecological contexts.

From this point of view, health must be interpreted as an element of the biographical as well as the social development. As a process, health is possible only if the individual, in a flexible and goal-oriented manner, is able to achieve the best possible coordination between inner and outer demands, at the same time ensuring a satisfactory continuity of self-experience (identity), and effecting his or her own realization by way of mutual agreement with and consideration for other interactors. Health is not a static, stable state, but a balance between various forces and demands that has to be continuously reviewed and readjusted in relation to the previous and continuing biography:

This makes health a leitmotiv of individuals' everyday activities, standing for the strength and energy required to structure life in close cooperation with others and, consequently, with the natural and social environment. Health has a subjective and socially developed space/time dimension. Both the subject and his or her life setting constitute the socioculturally developed locations of health. It should be possible that health is identifiable and can be experienced both in terms of the individual's subjective state and his or her life setting. If this linkage is not and/or cannot be established because it is not experienced in one and/or the other sphere, one could say that the subject's health is at risk. (Erben, Franzkowiak, & Wenzel 1986, p.69)

In this sense, physical, mental, and social health is only possible if an individual is able to develop constructive social relationships, become socially integrated, adapt his or her life design to the changing demands of the life setting, and, in so doing, express personal needs and derive a sense of fulfillment, while adapting this process to the biogenetic and physiological potentials and physical possibilities. If there is an adverse development in one domain, the effects may radiate to the other domains. For this reason, from a socialization-theoretical standpoint, it is necessary to undertake a comprehensive study of the physical, psychological, and social dimension of an individual's behavior for the purpose of identifying these forces that enhance or impair health.

Health is characterized by a productive subjective processing of societal conditions. A society's structural crises in employment and education, and in cultural values and social relations, lead to conflicts and frustrations with the result that, for a growing part of the population, an effective coping with subjectively experienced life stresses seems no longer possible. Conflicts at the workplace, in the family, in school, with friends, etc. mirror the complex and complicated living conditions of the highly individualized lifestyles of contemporary societies, characterized, as they are, by a high level of material wealth and a high risk of failure owing to manifold psychosocial stressors.

Chapter 6 Interventions: Strengthening Personal and Social Resources

In this final chapter, I want to examine the question of how the "welfare state" can

1. Organize conditions in the areas of work, home, education, human development, and recreation so that excessive strains on the social, psychological, and physical well-being of its citizens can be avoided as far as possible
2. At the same time reduce to a minimum the amount of delinquency, social disintegration, psychological disturbance, and physical illness

As a rule, the powers of interfering held by the state, the authoritative and administrative bodies, and other public organizations are subsumed under the collective term "intervention." The term describes activities of a helping, supportive, controlling, and corrective nature, whose aim is to intervene before deviance, disorders, and disease can develop fully. In other words, the goal is to avoid impending disorders ("preventive intervention"), to moderate existing disorders, and, if possible, to eliminate them ("correctional intervention").

Potential and Constraints of Intervention Strategies

State intervention in social conditions, including the areas of production and reproduction, is the classical object of a sociological theory of social politics (Kaufmann 1980, p.63). Kaufmann distinguishes three fundamental characteristics, stating that social politics always implies:

1. State intervention into a structured "social field"; the results of measures carried out by the state are partly dependent on the characteristics of this field
2. Intervention legitimated by considerations for individual well-being within specific target groups
3. Collective importance, since intervention is not legitimated by the satisfaction of an individual need, but by public interests

Within the last half century, in the Western states, the spectrum of social intervention has grown considerably, both in size and substance, and the number of areas regarded as being in need of intervention has greatly increased. It is only within the last few years that the growth of the welfare state appears to have reached its limits. Since the late 1980s, increases in the social budget have been curtailed in most of the industrial nations; the number of social political interventions and reform programs continue, at most, to grow at a slow pace. As a consequence, the influence of the state and its administrative bodies on the life course and personality development of the members of society has probably reached or even passed its zenith (Mayer & Müller 1986; Olk 1988).

Throughout the history of industrialization, the modern state has penetrated more and more areas of society. This is due to the state having essentially assumed responsibility for regulations concerning the organization of the economy, trade, transportation, communications, and working conditions, as well as vocational training and qualifications. At the same time, the state has assumed more responsibility for many aspects of the social welfare of its citizens, for example, poverty, unemployment, accidents, disablement, illness, old age, and ecological life space. The state acts as a controlling influence on the economic system, the employment sector, and the distribution of income, and as a consequence, secures the welfare of its citizens in numerous areas.

By implementing various measures, the state interferes with the way its citizens plan and conduct their daily lives. It intervenes, for example, by forbidding child labor, through legislation concerning school entry, the minimum age for marriage, retirement, and, indirectly, through legislation concerning taxes, family planning, career opportunities, etc. As a consequence, the state thereby defines almost all of the transitional stages in the life course, such as entry into employment, marriage, divorce, illness, disablement, and vocational training.

The idea of the welfare state — at least in the European tradition — is to increase the predictability and individual control of human existence through interventions of the kind already described and, as a consequence, to limit potential stress to a degree that does not exceed the capabilities of its citizens. In reducing economic constraints, the state also increases the potential for individual action and mobility, and thereby increases the likelihood that the individual will detach himself/herself from familial and other collective bonds. State intervention therefore has an integrating and a segregating effect on the way individuals organize their lives. On the one hand, the regulatory power of state institutions restricts the freedom to create individual lifestyles, on the other, the modern state at the same time offers possibilities that encourage individual decision making and individuality in general.

Types of Social Political Intervention

Kaufmann (1980, pp.66–84) divides the most important types of social and political intervention into the following four categories:

1. Measures to improve a person's legal status. Such measures entail protective rights (e.g., regarding employment of children) as well as the formation of individual and (subsequently) collective employment rights. For example, the following measures represent important types of social political intervention: the constitution of legal relationships such as strengthening consumer protection,

the modification of the rights of legal guardians, the introduction of the right to social security or to demand information.

2. Measures to improve a person's income. Such measures are aimed at a person's ability to satisfy his/her immediate material needs. Unter the conditions of a free-enterprise economy based on private capital, an individual's economic situation is essentially dependent on his/her access to a regular source of income. For persons who have access neither to earnings from assets nor from employment, measures are introduced which guarantee a basic income.

3. Measures to improve a person's material and social environment. The importance of such measures has increased within the last 30 to 40 years. They entail offers that necessitate a direct contact to the target person and that operate within his/her immediate vicinity. The benefits offered are either in the form of recreational space that can be actively utilized (e.g., parks, sports grounds, playgrounds), or as services which are directed toward the target persons (e.g., counseling, practical help). In order to reach the recipients and to be effective, the measures must be presented within the context of their immediate surroundings, the breadth of which varies according to the recipients' mobility. The state has increasingly assumed more responsibility in directly providing for social and material needs in these areas, a responsibility which has been legitimated by the term "quality of life." The effectiveness of such interventions depends on the extent to which the respective facilities and services are accessible to the target groups when needed.

4. Measures to improve a person's capabilities. The majority of such "pedagogical interventions" are aimed directly at persons who show a lack of social competence. The sociopolitical aim of these measures is the direct improvement of competence by way of educative, advisory, rehability, or informatory efforts. The central idea, therefore, is to convey knowledge and information to individuals in such a way as to increase their potential for participation. Pedagogical intervention can also be directed towards a third person who is involved with problem-ridden individuals. The focus hereby is primarily on supplementary education for those professional groups involved in the fields of education, counseling, and assistance.

Examples for these four modes of intervention in respect to typical measures and intended goals are as follows (Kaufmann 1980, p.85):

1. Typical measures:
   - Legal: provision of rights regarding protection, participation, complaints, jurisdiction, supervising bodies, rules regarding participatory activities
   - Economic: tax redistribution of inland revenue, financial support and compensation, tax concessions
   - Ecological: town and country planning, social planning, housing projects, financing of public facilities
   - Pedagogical: tuition based on curricular planning, provision of training and education, counseling, rehabilitation and information, support for self-help activities

2. Intended goals:
   - Legal: strengthen the legal situation of socially disadvantaged persons in regard to potential for participation
   - Economic: increase the available income of persons with insufficient means
   - Ecological: improve the quality and accessibility of environmental factors relevant to daily life
   - Pedagogical: increase the competence of persons in regard to legitimate possibilities of participation

Within the last three or four decades, there has been a continuing increase in demands and expectations in respect to state intervention; in particular, there has been a steady growth in demands on the state for political measures which are prophylactic or preventive in nature. The conditions within which large segments of the population live and work prove to be extremely detrimental. However, conventional measures of social political intervention do not guarantee permanent protection from social, psychological, and somatic impairment. As a consequence, social political measures which aim at increasing social resources and attempt to improve the conditions necessary for implementing measures of support and assistance are increasingly dependent on preventive measures that aim at the prophylactic avoidance of psychosocial pressures and health risks (Edelstein & Michelson 1986).

In recent years, there has been a continual increase in the expectations placed on preventive measures of intervention stemming from public institutions. The defense of basic human rights, that is, of personal freedom in respect to the state, has been increasingly interpreted as including the protection of civil rights: The state is expected to ensure that risks which are inherent in industrial societies do not interfere with personal freedom. Such demands on the state force it to extend its range of activities, often in such a way as to threaten traditional structures of the legal system, for in order to protect civil rights it is often necessary to curtail personal freedom.

Here we refer to the fact that an increase in administrative measures leads to a substantially broader interpretation of the term "basic human rights." The increase in demands for protection and prophylaxis can result in a growth of the controlling functions of the state. Not only is the state expected to shelter its citizens from disruptive social disorder and criminal acts, but additionally, demands are made on the state to deal with public health, collective acts of violence, economic deprivation, environmental pollution, etc. Accordingly, the actions of the state must be more anticipatory and comprehensive, rather than reactive and isolated. Expectations are no longer limited to the provision of assistance in cases of emergency and to corrective measures in legal areas. Instead, the state is expected to provide crisis prophylaxis, comprehensive guidance, and protection of civil liberties. Such demands may result in the state's being structurally overtaxed, as it frequently lacks the authority necessary for implementing prophylactic intervention (for example, with economy-oriented, job-protecting measures). However, it must attempt as far as possible to fulfill the increasing expectations on its sociopolitical imperative if it is to prevent social unrest and live up to its reputation as a welfare state.

Stimulation of Preventive and Self-Help Oriented Resources

It is quite evident that the limits of the traditional patterns of intervention on the part of the welfare state have been reached. This is partly due to the excessive strain on the state's finances, which results from its being given the responsibility for living conditions in general. In addition, the continued expansion of state influence cannot avoid having a counterproductive effect. In order to secure the personal freedom and the social demands of its citizens, the state would have to create institutions of control exceeding those of the present day. Administrative measures of prevention can only be expected to be successful when sufficient knowledge is available concerning the conditions and processes which result in disorders and impairments.

The more the preventive measures are directed towards "high-risk groups," the more comprehensive the information and data must be in order to facilitate a systematic identification of these groups. In the process of gathering such data, the danger increases that the voluntary principle in soliciting information will be transgressed or infringed upon. In the search for the causes of problem behavior, it is unavoidable that information from people's private lives is also accumulated, and that the future use of such information becomes open to abuse. As a consequence, state-controlled preventive measures can have negative side effects in the form of an invasion of people's privacy.

Therefore, for a variety of reasons, the expansion of traditional forms of social political intervention is neither expedient nor desirable. Within this context, the task of research must be to seek new forms of implementing help and support which avoid or prevent side effects such as a dependency, restrictions on personal freedom, and an increase in state control. This is only possible when both personal and social resources for dealing with concrete living conditions are strengthened; in other words, individual and collective capacities for coping with and mastering social reality must be strengthened, including the capacity for political articulation, representing self-interests, and self-organization (Hurrelmann, Kaufmann, & Lösel 1987).

As a prerequisite for such measures, numerous areas of governmental policies of intervention must be reorganized so that direct help is replaced by indirect, moderating help: immediate help is replaced by help which enables one to help oneself. Only such a policy of intervention can adequately live up to the standards of a democratic, pluralistic society which is structurally oriented towards encouraging and promoting individual competence.

This revised definition of intervention policy must be based on a realistic analysis of the functions of the welfare state. This implies recognizing the dual structure of the welfare state more clearly than has been the case so far — the formal and the informal sides, as well as the relationship between them. As Olk (1988) recently emphasized, formally organized systems of institutional help and support only make up one part of the help and support which is available and utilized in various situations and areas of daily life. The largest part of such supportive efforts takes place in the "informal regions" of the welfare state (Gottlieb 1983; Seidman 1983).

The degree of deprivation of individuals or social groups cannot be measured only in terms of their accessibility to public or semipublic social services; instead, it depends also on their accessibility to resources and facilities stemming from institutions of social support which operate on a voluntary basis and without state funding. We can distinguish between two distinct help sectors: a formal, organized help sector, which includes all state- and privately funded measures, and a nonprofessional help sector, which incorporates all nonfunded supportive measures in primary groups and voluntary organizations. The nonprofessional help sector can be divided again into two subgroups: all of the activities which take place within relationships in primary groups belong to the informal help sector, whereas the activities of the voluntary, nonprofit organizations belong to the voluntary help sector. Of course, this differentiation does not refer to two completely separate, independent sections of society; instead, we have here two highly interdependent components of a functional relationship. For the individual, this means that he/she is not involved in only one of these sectors; during the life course, each person receives (and, in part, produces) supportive measures within both sectors, as a rule, simultaneously (Olk 1988, p.6).

The rediscovery of these informal regions of the welfare state is strongly connected to the experiences of the past few years, in which the formal, regulatory mechanisms for the provision of assistance and support reached their limits. In terms of fiscal strength and political power, the welfare state is not in a position to expand its professional measures. The state-run health service, the government pension schemes, the educational system, the system of financial support for youths and socially underprivileged persons, etc. are only able to function in close cooperation with informal networks of assistance and support, both of which belong to the present-day "welfare state." In the face of the exaggerated expectations which exist in regard to administrative responsibility for public welfare, it is unavoidable that the informal measures be incorporated into governmental policy planning. Herein lies a danger that these informal areas will lose their political leverage. At the same time there exists a chance to reach broad and flexible political solutions which allow for a sensitive approach to the respective problem and risk areas of various individuals and groups.

Preventive and Corrective Interventions

The following is a description of forms of preventive and corrective interventions which attempt to adhere to the above-mentioned requirements. I hereby refer to the explanatory model based on socialization theory.

In the previous chapter, the thesis of a stage-by-stage process in the formation and development of disorders was presented. From the point of view of intervention theory, this necessitates designating the appropriate form of assisting personal and social resources for each of the stages in an attempt to interrupt this process. Usually, the terms "primary, secondary, and tertiary prevention" are utilized which were defined and established, for example, by Caplan and Grunebaum (1967) and Cowen (1983), and which are well-known in medical and psychiatric literature. However, we have modified this traditional terminology to a certain extent (Hurrelmann 1987a).

The term "preventive intervention" is used to describe all measures that are undertaken before behavior disorders become visibly manifest. Two types of preventive intervention can be identified: Firstly, those types which are directed towards improving the well-being and the social living conditions of individuals and groups in order to prevent the emergence of risk factors connected with disorders. These measures are aimed at preventing and protecting against personal and social factors which lead to disorders. Being anticipatory, they are, in the strict sense of the word "preventive"; in medical, psychiatric, and psychological literature they are usually characterized by the concept of "primary prevention." Secondly, preventive intervention includes all measures which are directed towards concrete, already visible risks for disorders. Here the aim is to diminish the anticipated effect of such risk factors by strengthening personal and social resources in order to reduce the likelihood of disorders. In this sense, the measures are directed towards preventing developments which have a high probability of resulting in disorders. If used in the strict sense, the term "secondary prevention," as used in the fields of medicine and psychiatry, describes these measures (Brandtstädter & von Eye 1982; Felner, Jason, Mortisugu, & Farber, 1983; Roberts & Peterson 1984).

It is important to note that both types or qualities of preventive intervention are directed towards strengthening individual resources in coping with risk factors as well as strengthening social resources, that is, the potential for support within the social environment. The goal of all preventive measures is to encourage and strengthen individual and social-environmental capacities which enable the individual to cope with stressful situations and critical events.

The term "corrective" intervention is reserved for those measures which are undertaken after disorders have been definitively identified. In an attempt to further differentiate these measures from preventive intervention, one could include the term "postventive intervention." Here, we also distinguish between two stages: The first stage of corrective intervention is directed towards disorders which are already manifest, whereby an attempt is made to diminish and reverse such disorders by implementing measures which strengthen personal and social resources. In this case, the measures are not of the aforementioned anticipatory (prophylactic) category; instead, they react to manifestations of delinquency, psychological disturbance or illness with the intention of "correcting" a person's behavior through various offers of a helping, remedial, advisory, and therapeutic nature. The second stage of corrective intervention comprises those measures which concentrate on mitigating a further intensification and consolidation of disorders. Here the accent is on reducing or avoiding the consequences of disorders and their negative effect on other areas of activity that accentuate developmental problems and establish a person's "career" of social deviance or problem behavior. The medical or psychiatric term "tertiary prevention" is used in a similar manner (Seidman 1983).

As in the case of measures of preventive intervention, here also the aim is to encourage individual or group competence and to strengthen social resources.

The terminology chosen here is preferred to "primary, secondary, and tertiary prevention," as it gives a more accurate description of the fact that the measures in question are, after all, intrusions, and as it avoids the inflationary use of the term "prevention." Common to both terminologies is the attempt to classify and designate measures according to the stage in the development of behavior disorders to which they are applied.

The previous statements clearly point out the importance of preventive intervention. All measures aimed at improving individual well-being, behavioral competence, self-esteem, and social living conditions — both material and nonmaterial — are of substantial importance for the success or failure of the entire process of socialization. Measures which are aimed at education, the family, youth services, employment, and legal policies, and which come in contact with existing personal and social capacities, are the most effective forms of social intervention (Frankenburg, Emde, & Sullivan 1985). In terms of costs, they also make ideal investments for society, for it is a well-proven fact that they make up only a fraction of the costs for subsequent treatment, remedies, therapy, and the control of habitual deviance, disorders, and their consequences, including drug abuse, crime, disablement, etc. (Apter 1978; Albee 1987; Burchard & Burchard 1987).

Intervention with Regard to Development

The above-mentioned approaches to intervention must be applied in a combined, coordinated process, if social, psychological, and physiological disorders are to be effectively dealt with. They must make allowances for the respective stages in the development of disorders, otherwise they remain one-sided and inappropriate. The goal of all intervention measures is to foster and strengthen the personal and social resources which enable individuals to cope with difficulties or stressful events during the life course.

We are dealing, therefore, with "individual competence promotion" and "social network promotion." In the last three decades, research into competence promotion has been given much greater priority. However, in the meantime, the social sciences have recognized the importance of the social environment for all attempts at intervention: Intervention can only be successful in combination with a reduction in the tensions and incongruity existing between biogenetic behavior and individual behavioral competence, on the one hand, and the demands of the social environment, on the other.

Current research shows that the intervention measures must be directed towards both poles of the aforementioned complex; they must be directed towards changing individual and social characteristics and resources. Measures which only concentrate on individuals must remain ineffective, as the individual capacities for acting and for coping with problems can only be influenced and altered within a social context. Having evolved in such a social context, that is, in a concrete social and ecological environment, this social and ecological environment must form an integral part of intervention policies if such policies are to have an effect on individual behavior.

If interventions are only directed towards the individual style of coping behavior, they may, as a result of not taking lifestyle factors into account and not being in touch with the prevailing social conditions, remain ineffective or, at best, lead to symptom displacement: Adolescents or adults who resort to smoking or alcohol consumption as a reaction to stress may become aware that such practices are a danger to health; as a consequence, however, they may shift the problem and become aggressive or depressive, resort to bad eating habits, or seek solace in other equally unhealthy forms of behavior (Silbereisen, Eyferth, & Rudinger 1986).

Disorder and illness must be regarded as societal phenomena that become visible in particular individuals: they "symptomize" themselves. Thus, problems are transposed from the societal level to the psychological and physical levels. They can be an expression of escape from an insolvable conflict and excessive stress, both of which can ultimately be traced back to social-structural conditions. Therefore, such problems can, in the long run, only be combated when the antecedent conditions of conflicts and stress are also tackled (Matarazzo et al. 1984).

Promotion of individual competence and social resources must be undertaken simultaneously due to the fact that well-being, personality development, and personal health are dependent on social, biological, and psychological factors; that is, on socioeconomic and natural living conditions, on genetic disposition, habitual, psychological components of behavior, present needs and interests, and on the individual's approach to work and leisure. Being conducive to good health, such factors must be incorporated into an overall structural context. From this vantage point, health promotion applies to the entirety of socioeconomic, legal, pedagogical, ecological, and biomedical interventions that are directed toward the accentuation and consolidation of capacities for employment, activity, the pursuit of pleasure, and the ability to make social contacts (Erben, Franzkowiak, & Wenzel 1986).

The advancement of personal and social resources for strengthening coping skills entails enabling all individuals to achieve a greater degree of autonomy over their environment and, as such, to make a contribution toward improving their own health. In order to achieve a state of physical, psychological, and social well-being, people must be able to satisfy their needs, to perceive and to realize their hopes and aspirations, and to cope with and influence their environment in a productive manner (Antonovsky 1987).

Advancement of Competence and Network Promotion

In this last section, potentials and constraints of strengthening personal and social resources will be discussed and illustrated with the aid of examples from various areas of activity. In accordance with the argumentation so far, and in an attempt to simplify the subject matter, a distinction will be made between the advancement and promotion of competence based on a strategy of strengthening personal resources, and the advancement and promotion of networks based on a strategy of strengthening social resources.

Promotion of Competence

Within this area, we can distinguish between three ideal types of intervention activity: education, counseling, and therapy.

Education

Education, being widely available, is the predominant mode of strengthening personal resources. Within industrial societies, the most important institutions for offering education are families, preschool facilities, schools, vocational training schemes, and higher educational and retraining institutions. The term "education" denotes the consciously planned, directive influence on individual personality development by means of another individual who is usually more knowledgeable and competent. In conveying knowledge, attitudes, and skills by systematically initiating learning steps, education aims at positively influencing the personality development of the recipient, strengthening his/her behavioral competency in various dimensions, and encouraging an autonomous process of acquisition by which an individual can have access to and adopt various capabilities (Tuma & Reif 1980).

The extensive transfer of responsibility for education to specialized institutions created particularly for this purpose is a typical aspect of industrial society. Here we have a concentration of the specific form of "pedagogical intervention" which aims at increasing behavioral capabilities by way of instructive activities. The necessity of pedagogical intervention which is implemented by means of education arises from the normative and practical interest that society shows towards the improvement of its members' behavioral capabilities, provided these capabilities are exercised within socially acceptable channels (Kaufmann 1980, p.80).

Pedagogical intervention represents a planned intrusion into the mediating process that takes place between societal demands on behavior and the behavioral competence of the individual members of society. Accordingly, such intervention operates between opposite poles of a functional relationship that takes place within socialization and that affects the process of personality growth which is determined by the acquisition and mastery of social and material living conditions.

The goal of all forms of pedagogical intervention must be to assist individuals in acquiring and utilizing behavior which enables them to effectively cope with social situations and life-events in a manner appropriate to their personality and environment.

The transference of knowledge and information is an integral part of every pedagogical intervention contained within the framework of education. The acquisition of knowledge and information within a systematic training context based on strict plans of education and instruction (curricula) takes place in school, whose official function is to convey knowledge as a basis for intellectual and social competence. Accordingly, in addition to conveying information, scholastic instruction entails the ability to utilize this knowledge as a matter of routine. Ideally, scholastic instruction conveys competencies which are relevant to areas within and beyond the school situation, that is, skills and abilities which are needed in daily life. Therefore, all instruction is essentially preventive in a direct sense, provided it is conceptionally oriented towards learning goals, pupil centered, and able to put psychological and pedagogical knowledge into practice.

As scholastic learning processes always take place within the context of the social interaction between teacher and student, intervention measures must take this interaction as their point of departure. In accordance with an analysis of causes that is based on socialization theory, appropriate pedagogical measures must take account of the social relationship between the adult and the child; in other words, they must concentrate on the form and content of interaction and communication between the teacher and the student. By concentrating on measures which are directed towards the individual, one soon reaches the limits of their effectivity. Instead, the entire social structure of the learning environment and the fundamental importance of the teacher-student relationship for the communication of knowledge must be incorporated into such measures. The learning context within the school, including its spatial aspects, and the specific demands of the curricula, must be regarded as a whole (Antonucci & Depner 1982; Apter 1982; Jason, Durlak, & Holton-Walker 1984; Elliot & Witt 1986).

This realization has been confirmed by the experience gained through preschool programs which suggest that the efforts of scholastic support and closer cooperation between kindergartens, preschool facilities, primary schools, and special schools should be increased. All reports of the long-term effects of the American Head Start and Follow Through programs, which in some cases have been carried out over a period of 15 years, show that the support ceases to be effective if the measures lack a firm foundation within the prevailing social environment (Schweinhart & Weikart 1987).

Counseling

In addition to conveying scholastic knowledge and educational skills through instruction, attention should be given to the type of intervention which is entailed in counseling. This type of intervention, which plays a key role in promoting competence, is, by virtue of its structural characteristics, protected against the dangers inherent in the controlling and disciplinary aspects of education. It is based on the principle of respecting and strengthening the addressee's behavioral autonomy: The recipients are treated as subjects who posses the potential for goal-oriented and rational actions. They are looked upon as self-responsible persons who, in principle, possess the capability and the will to make their own decisions.

Consequently, the basic principle of counseling entails the counselor having the ability to refrain from exerting influence other than to offer rational, emphatic arguments which are pragmatically oriented towards the goals, paths, and consequences of activities. Counseling is therefore based on the fundamental premise that the client is able to make decisions and to use reasoning. This premise distinguishes counseling from those types of ecological, legal, or economic interventions that involve a "manipulation" of living conditions and that, at least occasionally, are carried out without obtaining the consent of the recipient (Rutter 1980).

Let us take youth counseling as an example. Here, the aim of the counseling process must be to assist the adolescent in securing the status of an autonomous, competent, and self-sufficient individual, without resorting to uncontrolled manipulation. Counseling, therefore, offers temporary help in unravelling and coping with stressful situations and environmental conditions in cases where persons are in difficulty as a result of lacking the full capacity to deal with their problems. The counselor must employ his/her competence in such a way that it contributes toward the establishment or reestablishment of the adolescent's ability to act. The counselor must possess enough professional competence to enable the individual to rediscover and redevelop capabilities which have been retarded or weakened. From an interaction-theory perspective, counseling must have the structure of a "discourse" in which the counselor and the client make a concerted attempt to find a solution to problems while maintaining a relationship based on mutual respect.

The fundamental principle of youth counseling must be to avert a consolidation of already established processes of deviance and disorders, and to activate recognizable possibilities of correcting behavior. Both aims can be accomplished by introducing new definitions and interpretations of situations, suggestions on how to reduce self-restraints, and other similar measures which contribute toward self-identity and self-control. The counselor must recognize behavior disorders and impairments in personality development as being expressions of the fact that the adolescent's attempts at coping with the social environment and its demands do not conform to the expectations of the environment and/or to his/her own needs (Roberts & Peterson 1984).

The counselor, therefore, must, on the one hand, concentrate on strengthening and promoting the adolescent's behavioral competence so that he/she can effectively cope with the demands of the social environment (e.g., school) and avoid getting into difficulties. On the other hand, competencies must be encouraged that enable him/her to influence and change the social environment through increased participation (Albee 1987).

Therapy

The proximity of counseling to therapy has been emphasized repeatedly in the literature, and there is evidence to suggest that both terms should be used synonymously. For example, therapeutic techniques such as client-centered therapy and other forms of communicative therapy border on classical concepts of counseling. It is, however, more efficacious to regard counseling and therapy as two poles in a continuum of various types of intervention with varying characteristics and permeable borders.

Common to both forms is that the goal — behavioral change — can only be achieved when client (advice-seeker) and counselor (advice-giver) are in agreement. Counseling and therapy can only be successful when they are directed towards the existing personal and social resources of the client. A counselor or therapist can only support personality development by supplying information, possibilities, and resources which have been lacking, and by assisting in restoring and redirecting resources that have been falsely interpreted or inadequately utilized.

In the long term, a therapist, or a counselor, cannot be a substitute for behavior which must come from the client; instead, the client must be viewed as an independent and self-responsible partner to whom support can be given in his/her attempts to achieve his/her own goals and to gain more understanding within a process of increasing self-knowledge and self-control. This support must augment existing potential and subjective theories of day-to-day living. Accordingly, as with counseling, therapy represents a kind of dialogue by consensus, a process whereby, in a mutual effort to reach agreement in assessing potential solutions, therapist and client undertake a combined search for the most suitable solutions to particular problems. It is important that the client be able to recognize the problem of his/her own accord, to utilize the aid of the therapist in order to perceive it accurately, and finally, to contribute to its solution through his/her own self-efforts.

Differences exist between counseling and therapy above all in the point of departure, duration, and methods. The main function of counseling involves the transfer of information and assessments, the use of which enables the client to overcome difficulties in orientation and to improve the informational basis on which subjectively complex, momentary decisions are made. The central aim of therapy is to instigate and structure a process by which habitual behavioral symptoms are recognized as being inadequate coping strategies and which are to be reduced or made superfluous. When a person is in a difficult situation or in an emergency whose source does not lie within the person and which can be immediately tackled, counseling is expedient. By contrast, therapy proves necessary when a person is involved in an intense and long-lasting psychological conflict with which he/she is unable to cope (Erikson 1959; Cullinan, Epstein, & Lloyd 1983; Garmezy & Rutter 1983; Lauth 1983).

The counseling situation is, therefore, more of a consultatory arrangement in which information is passed on, and where, as a rule, a relatively brief contact suffices in dealing with the situation. Within therapy, on the other hand, a treatment situation is required in which verbal and other symbolic exchanges governed by rules are utilized and, as a consequence, the usual behavior patterns of daily life are suspended. Whereas during counseling, a restricted, sectional, and short-term interaction between counselor and client is possible, therapy necessitates a more comprehensive and longer-lasting contact, due to the utilization of revelational procedures which, for example, attack existing defense mechanisms.

Promotion of Social Networks

All of the above-mentioned methods of strengthening personal resources and of promoting individual competence are measures which prove effective in the areas of prevention and correction. However, their limits are evident: They represent a „removing the symptom" approach, inasmuch as they are simply manifestations of individual measures of coping with conflicts and problems which have their origins in part, if not in sum, in areas external to the person involved. Consequently, they must be instigated in combination or, at least, in connection with measures which strengthen social resources.

Questions must be asked of research into intervention as to how the relationship networks in various social areas should be put into practice, what relevance they have for self-image and coping capacity, and, above all, how those social processes that have a positive effect on networks can be strengthened.

As a rule, theoretical analyses in this area take as their point of departure the most traditional type of network: the family. Even within conditions of change, the family proves to have the greatest importance in the development of personality. No other social institution surpasses it in terms of duration, intensity, and suggestibility. Nevertheless, in many ways, the social position of the family within present-day industrial society is endangered. As shown above, today's families are systems which are small and vulnerable to disturbance, and the percentage of marriages (and other cohabitant relationships) which remain childless is on the increase. Families today are extremely dependent on support in dealing with their responsibilities, above all, in raising children and in caring for family members who are old and, in many cases, infirm. They are, therefore, in urgent need of offers of social resources in order to cope with intrafamilial, stressful events, and also, to be able to at least partly perform those tasks which are difficult to transfer to society's formal institutions.

Fostering Family Networks

In organizing internal processes such as care, attentiveness, and support, as well as child rearing and the provision of nourishment, the family gains social resources through the process of interaction with the social environment. In fulfilling its social functions, the family is dependent on utilizing the services offered by external social systems. If these services are lacking or inadequate, a crisis can develop in the systems which regulate social interactions and economic security within the family (Sussman & Steinmetz 1987).

Kaufmann, Herlth, and Strohmeier (1980, p.103) distinguish three groups of external social resources which the family depends on:

1. Ecological resources constitute, on the one hand, the spatial, material conditions within the family environment; in this sense, they incorporate the provision of living space and of long-term and short-term consumer goods. On the other hand, ecological resources include social aids and services which are supplied by the social environment (e.g., repair services, possibilities of delegating household chores such as laundering and cooking), information services, assistance from informal networks such as neighbourly help, and public services such as counseling, or education.
2. Economic resources refer to the financial means which a family must make available within its environment in order to satisfy its need for ecological and cultural resources.
3. Cultural resources entail the participation of individuals in the entirety of forms of collective knowledge that are available within society. Participation in public knowledge establishes an orientation towards activity in general, acts as a stabilizing factor on motivation, and thus permanently assures the performance of daily activities.

The sum of these social resources which exist within the family environment, that is, public and private aids, support, and services, influence the family's internal structure (McCubbins, Sussman, & Patterson 1984). The resources must be available in sufficient measure and be utilized by the family in a flexible manner appropriate to the situation in which they are applied if they are to contribute to the family's efforts to fulfill its responsibilities for self-maintenance, self-care, and childrearing. Social services must be introduced in such a way as to ensure maximum efficacy and utilization, and to support and strengthen processes within the family that contribute towards the well-being of its individual members.

The likelihood that a family will utilize the available political resources depends to a great extent on the family's social and economic situation, its physical environment, and, above all, on its degree of integration within the local community. Due to the dependence of the family members' psychological, physical, and social well-being on their active participation, political measures must come into contact with the social situation of the family and increase the participation of its individual members. In other words, social well-being is dependent on the type and degree of integration within the relationship network of the social environment — particularly the neighborhood — and on the possibilities for participating in political decisions within the community (Albee 1987; Cochran 1987).

In industrial societies, family policy should concentrate on and limit itself to providing resources for the family, and ways and means with which such resources can be implemented. In a democratic society, the goal of such a policy cannot be to go beyond this aim and to dictate concrete patterns of behavior and lifestyles, or to stipulate the conditions under which such resources are to be given. If family social policies are to be effective and justifiable, they must resist the temptation to control the family members' behavior in accordance with particular political priorities. Even incentive programs of the kind described above, do, of course, exert a subtle control. They can, however, be justified, as long as they retain their voluntary character and are directed towards strengthening the potential contained in the environment of the family as well as the individual family member's ability to participate in the environment. Essentially, this involves activities which create a broad basis for cultural, community-oriented work which is not governed by regulations. The aim of such culturally supportive programs is to make public life more transparent — both within the community and the society at large — and, as a consequence, more interesting for the individual family member (Simmons 1981; Erben, Franzkowiak, & Wenzel 1986, p.112).

Strengthening Participatory Potential

The dilemma of most family-oriented intervention programs can only be overcome if such programs are based on participation: As a rule, the need for social intervention — in particular, the need for financial and social resources provided by institutions of social aid — is only acknowledged when a family is in a situation of material and social deprivation. In many cases, support such as social assistance, additional educative programs, nutritional aid, rent supplements, and additional support in the areas of child-care and health are only provided when it can be proven that families are completely lacking in resources of their own. Therefore, in order to qualify for state support, such families must show an extreme lack of means and facilities. In a sense, parents and children must demonstrate their inadequacy and lack of social integration in order to gain access to social services, with the result that they often become dependent on such services.

Such conditions, which are ethically unacceptable, and, in terms of family-oriented intervention, politically unproductive, must be surmounted. The goal must be to assist the family's social environment, the supportive network, in preventing the family from entering an unfavorable economic and social situation. This entails organizing the potential for support contained in the environment, as well as the family's self-organizing ability.

This is known as the concept of "empowering": The aim of intervention is to strengthen the family members' social network through precise, well-planned measures which enable them to articulate and defend their own interests (Cochran 1987, p.108). The central aim, therefore, is to enable individuals to influence other people and organizations to their own advantage. In this way, the process of subordination and humiliation which normally forms a basis for the mobilization of social support can be avoided. In this sense, the concept of "empowering" is directed against the "deficit model," which is implicated in most present-day strategies of social intervention. It makes allowances for the structural, economic, ecological, and cultural disadvantages of large numbers of families. These disadvantages can only be eradicated by participatory policies that are directed at these structural characteristics and that strengthen the self-help potential contained in such families.

Increasingly, arguments which emphasize structural components of intervention and a strategy of "network support" are also being proposed by social-medical and social-psychological research. The relationship between stressful situations and coping behavior, on the one hand, and psychosomatic symptoms and illness as a reaction to stress, on the other, has been recognized for quite some time. However, it was not until recently that the importance of the social context and structure of social relationships in regard to the occurrence of illness received attention. In the meantime, the promotion of social networks within the family, neighborhood, school, and employment situations and their relationship to formal and informal health care has increasingly become a subject of discussion.

From this viewpoint, the goal of intervention is to discover, alleviate, or eliminate environmental risk factors, and to strengthen factors which are conducive to good health. The strategy of network support could prove to be an effective instrument in implementing this new philosophy of physical and mental health. The term "network support" is used to describe measures which (a) serve to support, relieve, and mobilize existing networks within the family, employment situation, and community, and (b) are directed towards initiating or supporting new network elements, for example, the establishment of self-help groups or organizations. The strategy of network support is unspecific, the aim being to improve general conditions of public health. This strategy proves to be optimal, as it is directed towards the expansion of health resources, without making stipulations as to the use and effectivity of the resources during individual application (Badura 1983, p.42).

Network support also includes flexible measures of advisory activities which, within the framework of loosely structured models of counseling, attempt to supplement traditional therapeutic, client-centered methods of family counseling through procedures oriented towards the community and the conditions of daily life. From a "network perspective," achieving the goal of environmental participation entails attempting the following (Keupp & Röhrle 1987):

1. Strengthening existing support systems within the immediate vicinity of the family (relatives, neighborhood, circle of friends) and incorporating the respective reference persons, as "natural counselors", into the helping process
2. Establishing alternative networks for the family members in the case where utilizing the family network is not possible or desirable
3. Transforming the counseling institution into a meeting place which can serve as an additional social network for problem families
4. Transcending the boundaries of the traditional framework of counseling and carrying out extensive parts of the counseling process within the family's home environment

Emphasis should hereby be placed on the type of access first mentioned, that is, on the attempt to bring a new quality of support and assistance into the family's social networks. The procedures must be carried out with caution and sensitivity;

after all, such procedures, although aimed at strengthening the internal organization of the family, do represent an intrusion by an external power into the family's daily life.

Of course, in addition to strengthening "network counseling," the traditional fields of counseling that are directed towards the family and child rearing, that is, parental and educational advisory services, must also be reinforced. Due to the complex demands facing parents in day-to-day life, the coping abilities of a growing number of parents are evidently being stretched to their limits. Parents' personal and partnership problems result in insecurity, loss of authority, contact difficulties, and in the abuse, maltreatment, and neglect of their children. Such behavior is deeply rooted in the structure of the relationships of the respective families (Garbarino, Schellenbach, & Sebes 1986). The increasing pressure on parents to provide their children with a good education in order to secure the parents' social and professional status acts as an additional stress factor.

In this field, general parental education proves effective, such as information about questions of child rearing and adolescence which take the form of evening classes, group work, circulars, family recreation, and similar such measures. In the event that problem situations arise, counseling and supportive measures for parents prove necessary. All of these measures are of an explanatory and informative nature; they attempt to strengthen parents' competence in regard to the process of their children's socialization, and to offer such parents orientation and help in planning and making decisions. In this sense, network promotion is inseparable from competence promotion.

Comprehensive Health Promotion

Corresponding to current thought in health research, a comprehensive approach which goes beyond the bounds of individual-oriented intervention can also be observed in other social and political areas. In accordance with the concept of "health promotion," changes have taken place within youth work, scholastic and extracurricular education, and vocational training. In addition to the promotion of individual competence, emphasis is being placed on the importance of environmental factors, above all, with respect to health-relevant behavior of both adolescents and adults, and to intervention measures that are aimed directly at this behavior.

The main impetus for such comprehensive concepts of health promotion stems from the experience gained within the confines of health-promoting programs that were sponsored by public health and were of a purely empirical, informative, and explanatory nature. They adhered mostly to a pedagogically based program of individual measures aimed at encouraging behavior that was conducive to good health. This concept of health-promoting behavior was given priority among preventive strategies operating in the areas of youth services and education. However, the success of such informative pedagogical measures remains limited due to the fact that knowledge and information are factors which can change well-established, social patterns of behavior only under certain conditions (Perry & Jessor 1985).

However, it is not always appropriate for a person to behave in a manner which is favorable to good health. As we have seen, behavior which endangers health is closely tied up with routine daily life and is part of a general lifestyle. Tobacco and alcohol consumption, for example, can have a compensatory function in stressful situations at work or during leisure. Therefore, behavior, which, from an objective point of view, is damaging to health, can also have a stress-reducing function in respect to other risk factors. In other words, behavior is not necessarily guided by cognitive knowledge regarding its negative effect on health (Wills 1985). Drug consumption is frequently a symptom of a more profound coping crisis. As a consequence, most drug-prevention programs, being based on informative and explanatory measures, prove to be basically inadequate in their approach. They ignore the social factors of health-damaging behavior as well as the psychological and social significance which such ostensibly health-damaging behavior has for the individual.

For measures to be effective, it is important that the entire social environment be incorporated into the health-promoting measures in such a way that such measures are introduced within the context of the adolescent's or adult's familial, scholastic/occupational, and other social relationships. The fundamental question is as follows: How can the desires for independence, intensive experiences, companionship, personal relationships, self-knowledge, accomplishment, and self-confidence be satisfied? Drug use enables one to make an impression on the social environment to the extent that these desires appear to have been fulfilled. It can only be replaced when alternative forms of satisfying such desires are made available. In this respect, the style of communication and relationships within the family and at school are frequently regarded by adolescents as restrictive and are apparently inadequate for such a task. Adolescents seek possibilities for communication which extend beyond the boundaries set by the institutions of socialization. Health-promoting measures must therefore attempt to support adolescents in their efforts to find an individual lifestyle.

Mechanic and Hansell (1988) point out that we know a great deal about how adults assess their health status, but much less about such assessments among young people. In their opinion, a general self-assessment of health is useful because it is among the best predictors of health-related behavior:

The self-assessment of health is an active process involving general cognitive and emotional strategies for understanding the self; physical symptoms are simply one possible building block of an overall self-assessment of health that may have several components. Particular physical symptoms may be given prominence or may be viewed as peripheral compared with other aspects of the self and the social environment. Understanding the determinants of such assessments will help us understand why individuals with comparable physical morbidity and physical impairment vary so widely in their levels of social disability and in their use of medical services. (Mechanic & Hansell 1988, p.365)

Young people typically have relatively low rates of serious physical morbidity. They report better health status than adults. However, in the relative absence of chronic health problems, adolescents construct self-assessments of health based on other, more salient criteria. They assess their physical health in terms of their competence in important areas of adolescent life and their sense of psychological well-being. Self-assessments of better health are influenced directly by higher levels of competence, as measured by grades in school and participation in sports and exercise, and by greater psychological well-being, as indicated by lower levels of depressed mood.

> For adolescents, health is truly a social concept in the sense intended by the World Health Organization definition, and reflects competence in age-appropriate activities. If we form attitudes about ourselves by observing our own action..., then adolescents may conclude that they are healthy in part because they are active and competent. (Mechanic & Hansell 1988, p.371)

As a consequence, health-promoting programs that aim at correcting behavior must incorporate the various facets of the social environment and the enmeshment of sociocultural and economic living conditions with health factors. Intervention can only be expected to succeed when health promotion is understood as an aid to coping with daily problems, and when the factors which play a part in the coping process are included (Franzkowiak 1986). The organization of individual behavior, which can also be regarded as the avoidance of risk-prone habits, seems, as a prerequisite, to demand that the individual have a chance to actively shape and control his/her social environment. A student, for example, may be prepared to refrain from risk behavior (smoking, drug-use), when the school system, and the school attended, offer the opportunity to reach the aspired goal and thereby avoid experiencing despair in attending school. According to this premise, individuals will be able to refrain from health-endangering behavior only after individual interests, for example, at work, school, or in the community, have been taken care of. Here, prevention and political work can be linked together.

Risks to health are also influenced by environmental factors and by the entire constellation of sociostructural living conditions. Here, individual behavior plays a comparatively small role. Intervention of a preventive and correctional nature must consider the prevailing environmental conditions that lead to disorders, as well as the specific individual reactions and symptoms that are connected with the latter. Thus, school, leisure activities, friendships, employment, housing and traffic facilities fall within the area of political intervention efforts (Wiley & Camacho 1980).

Health Promotion in Adolescence

In closing, the points made so far will be exemplified within the context of comprehensive health promotion among adolescents. This refers to preventive intervention that is directed towards the social, psychological, and physical well-being of adolescents within school, family, leisure, and employment situations.

Within the school situation, what is primarily needed is a comprehensive empirically based pedagogical concept, which, in addition to scholastic elements, incorporates elements of social pedagogy. Within this area, the goal of such measures must be to allow school to become a stimulating component of the adolescents' daily life, and which serves to create space for important experiences and contributes towards personal development. The school must be able to offer facilities for work and training in various areas of learning that can be perceived as important and worthwhile by the adolescent. In this sense, a good school is a social situation which has a preventive effect on behavior disorders and antisocial behavior.

Of course, being an institution of organized education, the school plays a leading role in transposing informative programs of health education into practice that establish connections between health and work, environment, culture, and social structures, and that accumulate information about factors which are detrimental to health. In addition to tuition of a cognitive and informative nature, stimulation in the areas of music, art, and sports plays an important role. In school, body consciousness and sensual experience can be developed and incorporated into a comprehensive pedagogical concept of health promotion.

In terms of familial areas of activity, intervention measures must ensure that an adequate degree of economic security and cultural stimulation is provided, if, for example, adolescents are to be discouraged from using health-impairing drugs. Satisfactory parent-child relationships are the prerequisites for such a goal. Thus, active preventive measures must enable the family to remain a reliable reference group in situations of economic or psychological crisis. The family is the most important informal source of health education during childhood and adolescence; it also forms basic attitudes to future health-relevant behavior. Through activities in day-to-day life, such as dental care, diet, medical treatment, hygiene, vaccination, clothing, sex education, accident prevention, etc., the foundations are laid for concepts of body consciousness, a lifestyle conducive to good health, and self-esteem.

In regard to leisure activities, situations must be created which offer adolescents experiences and encounters which distract them from the temptations of consumerism, and which dissuade them from participating in delinquent group behavior or other dangerous activities. Herein lies a dilemma, in that adolescents have access to many social and material possibilities but, at the same time, lack real challenges and means of satisfying their interests and needs due to the superficial satisfaction offered by present-day mass media and a consumer-oriented society. Such fulfillment often entails a false sense of adventure and experience; there exists a lack of real challenges and personal experiences which enable a young person to utilize his/her physical prowess and psychological and social competence.

Situations are lacking in which noncommercial, unorganized, unsupervised, and "nonpedagogical" activities can take place which enable adolescents to test their potentials and limitations, and in which they are free to "experiment" with the limits set by laws and conventions, without fear of sanctions. Our highly civilized and highly structured environment leaves little room for such "free space." Herein lies a great challenge to youth work and youth support; an attempt must be made to "artificially" recreate such free spaces. In other words, social resources must be created which stimulate and support a healthy development of personality and which have ceased to exist as a result of the organization of daily life that is typical of industrial societies.

In health promotion, attention must be paid to the fact that social relationships which are experienced as being supportive directly affect physical, psychological, and social well-being, and are prerequisites for overcoming stressful living conditions. For this reason, support in establishing and maintaining social relationships is an integral part of youth work and youth counseling. Adolescents must be given the opportunity to articulate and fulfill their own needs through self-help groups, participation in community projects, and through living in groups which have common goals (Coleman 1961). The development of adolescents' competence at self-organizing — as individuals and as groups — necessitates offering resources and indicating paths by which contacts and employment possibilites can be reached (Hildebrandt 1987, p.91). In this area, new methods must be introduced even though social structures and conditions only permit limited possibilities.

In the area of employment, network-oriented health promotion must aim at giving the term "work" a positive connotation that suggests the possibility of creating something worthwhile, of making a contribution to society, of developing and creating products, of expressing oneself as an individual, and of transposing ideas and thoughts into concrete actions. Therefore, the efforts should not only be directed towards protection against physical and biochemical risks at places of work. The working conditions must be formed according to the psychosocial possibilities and needs of the employees. Increasing individual responsibility and information about occupational health hazards, as well as encouraging supportive relationships among work colleagues, have a positive effect on employees' health. In addition, working conditions must be created which promote a sense of identity with the product of work.

Above all, in present-day youth work, the goal must be to create possibilities of youth employment and to tackle unemployment. Even in our so-called leisure society, self-concept and prestige are essentially determined by one's occupation. Society places adolescents in enormous difficulties by not being able to guarantee training or employment on completion of school. It thereby destroys the necessary amount of confidence in the future, which adolescents are dependent on during this phase of life. For decades, the entry into a field of occupation has, in addition to marriage and starting a family, been a decisive and symbolic step into adulthood. If this step cannot be taken, we deprive adolescents of the social foundations of healthy personality development (Hurrelmann & Engel 1989).

As this discussion shows, health must be regarded as an integral part of a person's entire development. It must be incorporated into comprehensive concepts of support that address the problems of the environment, hygiene, eating habits, social security, orientation towards the future, lifestyle, and self-concept. According to this understanding, health promotion is an interdisciplinary area which includes medicine, biology, epidemiology, psychology, psychiatry, sociology, and pedagogy. As yet, no integrated system of health promotion exists that incorporates health education, health information, and health counseling; instead, these fields of practical work are divided into numerous areas. It is conceivable that the various activities could be brought together if, as a first step, community-based health counseling institutions, health bureaus, and medical doctors should cooperate with, for example, family counseling services, child guidance clinics, social work in schools, adolescent counseling, prenatal clinics, drug counseling services, and crisis services (Caplan 1974; Antonovsky 1979; Simmons 1981).

Health promotion cannot be supported and maintained solely by the health sector. Rather, it demands a coordinated effort on the part of all those responsible in the fields of education and social services, in nongovernmental and self-organized associations and initiatives, in institutions responsible for community affairs, and, finally, in industry and the media. Health promotion entails more than just medical and social services; it must be actively pursued at all levels of sociopolitical activity.

References

Achenbach, T.M., & McConaughy, S.H. (1987) *Empirically based assessment of child and adolescent psychopathology*. Beverly Hills: Sage

Albee, G.W. (1987) Powerlessness, politics, and prevention. In Hurrelmann, K., Kaufmann, F.X. & Lösel, F. (Eds.): *Social intervention: Potential and constraints*. Berlin: De Gruyter, 37–52

Aneshensel, C.S., & Fredrichs, R.R. (1982) Stress, support and depression: Longitudinal causal model. *Journal of Community Psychology, 10,* 363–376

Antonovsky, A. (1979) *Health, stress, and coping*. San Francisco: Jossey Bass

Antonovsky, A. (1987) *Unraveling the mystery of health*. San Francisco: Jossey Bass

Antonucci, T.C., & Depner, C.E. (1982) *School support and informal helping relationships*. New York: Academic Press

Apter, S.A. (Ed.) *Focus on prevention*. Syracuse: Syracuse University Press

Apter, S.J. (1982) *Troubled children, troubled systems*. New York: Pergamon

Bachman, J.G., Johnston, L.D., & O'Malley, P. (1981) Smoking, drinking, and drug use among American High School students. *American Journal of Public Health, 71,* 59–67

Bachman, J.G., O'Malley, P.M., & Johnston, L.D. (1982) *Youth in transition*. Vol.7. Ann Arbor: University of Michigan Press

Bachman, J.G., Johnston, L.D., O'Malley, P.M., & Humphrey, R.H. (1988) Explaining the recent decline in marijuana use: Differentiating the effects of perceived risks, disapproval, and general lifestyle factors. *Journal of Health and Social Behavior, 29,* 92–112

Badura, B. (Ed.) (1981) *Soziale Unterstützung und chronische Krankheit*. Frankfurt: Suhrkamp

Badura, B. (1983) *Sozialepidemiologie in Theorie und Praxis*. Europäische Monographien zur Forschung in Gesundheitserziehung. Bd. 5, 29–48

Baethge, M. (1989) Individualization as hope and as disaster. In Hurrelmann, K., & Engel, U. (Eds.): *The social world of adolescents*. Berlin: De Gruyter, 37–52

Baltes, P.B., Featherman, D.L., & Lerner, R.M. (Eds.) (1986) *Life span development and behavior. Vol. 7*. Hillsdale: Erlbaum

Bandura, A. (1977) Self-efficacy. Toward a unifying theory of behavioral change. *Psychological Review, 84,* 191–215

Beck, U. (1986) *Risikogesellschaft*. Frankfurt: Suhrkamp

Berkman, L.F. (1985) The relationship of social networks and social support to morbidity and mortality. In Cohen, S., & Syme, S.L. (Eds.): *Social support and health*. New York: Academic

Berkman, L.F., & Breslow, L. (1983) *Health and ways of living: The Alameda County study*. New York: Oxford University Press

Berman, A.L. (1986) Helping suicidal adolescents: Needs and responses. In Corr, C.A., & McNeil, J.N. (Eds.): *Adolescence and death*. New York: Springer, 151–164

Biddle, B., Bank, B.J., & Marlin, M.M (1980) Parental and peer influence on adolescents. *Social Forces, 58,* 1057–1079

Bleidick, U. (1987) *Rahmenbedingungen für die Integration Behinderter*. Hamburg. Research paper

Borman, K.M. (Ed.) (1982) *The social life of children in a changing society*. Hillsdale: Erlbaum

Bourdieu, P. (1984) *Distinctions. A social critique of the judgement of taste*. London: Routledge

Boyce, W.T. (1985) Social support, family relations, and children. In Cohen, S., & Syme, S.L. (Eds.): *Social support and health*. Orlando: Academic Press

Brandtstädter, J., & Eye, A.v. (Hg.) (1982) *Psychologische Prävention*. Bern: Huber

Bräutigam, W. & Christian, P. (1986) *Psychosomatische Medizin*. Stuttgart: Thieme

Brim, O.G., & Kagan, J. (1980) *Constancy and change in human development*. Cambridge: Harvard University Press

Bronfenbrenner, U. (1979) *The ecology of human development*. Cambridge: Harvard University Press

Brown, G.W., & Harris, T. (1978) *Social origins of depression. A study of psychiatric disorder in women*. London: Tavistock

Bundesministerium für Jugend, Familie und Gesundheit (1987) *Daten des Gesundheitswesens*. Stuttgart: Kohlhammer

Burchard, J.D., & Burchard, S.N. (Eds.) (1987) *Prevention of delinquent behavior*. Beverly Hills: Sage

Butler, N.R., & Corner, B.B. (Eds) (1984) *Stress and disability in childhood*. Bristol: Wright

Caplan, G (1974) *Support systems and Community Mental Health*. New York: Academic

Caplan, G., & Grunebaum, H. (1967) Perspectives on primary prevention. A review. *Archives in Genetic Psychiatry, 17*, 331–346

Cassel, J. (1975) Social science in epidemiology: Psychosocial processes and "stress" theoretical formulations. In Struening, E.L., & Guttentag, M. (Eds.): *Handbook of evaluation research, Vol. 11*. Beverly Hills: Sage, 537–549

Chess, S., & Thomas, A. (1986) *Temperament in clinical practice*. New York: Guilford

Chiriboga, D.A., & Cutler, L. (1980) Stress and adaptation: Life span perspectives. In: Poon, L.W. (Ed.): *Aging in the 1980s*. Beverly Hills: Sage, 347–362

Clausen, J.A. (1984) Mental illness and the life course. In Baltes, P.B., & Brim, O.G. (Eds.): *Life span development and behavior. Vol. 6*. New York: Academic, 203–242

Clausen, J.A. (1986a) Early adult choices and the life course. *Zeitschrift für Sozialisationsforschung und Erziehungssoziologie, 6*, 313–320

Clausen, J.A. (1986b) *The life course*. Englewood Cliffs: Prentice Hall

Clausen, J.A. (1987) Health and the life course: Some personal observations. *Journal of Health and Social Behavior, 28*, 337–344

Cobb, S. (1976) Social support as a moderator of life stress. *Psychosomatic Medicine, 38*, 300–314

Cochran, M. (1987) Empowering families: An alternative to the deficit model. In Hurrelmann, K., Kaufmann, F.X., & Lösel, F. (Eds.): *Social intervention: Potential and constraints*. Berlin: De Gruyter, 105–120

Cohen, S., & Syme, S.L. (Eds.) (1985) *Social support and health*. Orlando: Academic

Coleman, J.S. (1961) *The adolescent society*. New York: Free Press

Coleman, J.C. (1980) *The nature of adolescence*. New York: Methuen

Condry, J.C. (1984) Gender identity and social competence. *Sex Roles, 11*, 485–511

Conrad, P., & Schneider, J.W. (1980) *Deviance and medicalization*. New York: Pergamon

Cooper, C.L., & Payne, R. (Eds.) (1980) *Current concerns in occupational stress*. New York: Wiley

Corson, S.A. & Corson, E.O. (1983) Biopsychogenetic stress. In Selye, H. (Ed.): *Selye's guide to stress research. Vol 2*. New York: Von Nostrand

Cowen, E.L. (1983) Primary prevention in mental health: Past, present, and future. In Felner, R.D., Jason, L.A., Mortisugu, J., & Farber, S.S. (Eds.): *Preventive psychology*. New York: Pergamon, 11–25

Cullinan, D., Epstein, M.H, & Lloyd, J. (1983) *Behavior disorders of children and adolescents*. Englewood Cliffs: Prentice Hall

Diekstra, R.F.W., & Hawton, K. (Eds.) (1987) *Suicide in adolescence*. Dordrecht: Nijhoff

Dillon, K.M., Minchoff, B., & Baker, K.H. (1985) Positive emotional states and enhancement of the immune system. *International Journal of Psychiatry in Medicine, 15*, 13–18

Dodge K.A. (1986) A social information processing model of social competence in children. In: Perlmutter, M. (Ed.): *Minnesota symposium on child psychology. Vol. 18*. Hillsdale: Erlbaum, 77–125

Dohrenwend, B.P. (1975) Sociocultural and sociopsychological factors in the genesis of mental disorders. *Journal of Health and Social Behavior, 16,* 365–392

Dohrenwend, B.P., & Dohrenwend, B.S. (1981) Socio-environmental factors and psychopathology. *American Journal of Community Psychology, 9,* 128–164

Dohrenwend, B.P., Dohrenwend, B.S., Gould, M.S., Link, B., Neugebauer, R., & Wunsch-Hitzig, R. (1980) *Mental illness in the United States: Epidemiological estimates.* New York: Praeger

Dohrenwend, B.S., & Dohrenwend, B.P. (1974) *Stressful life events: Their nature and effects.* New York: Wiley

Donovan, J.E., & Jessor, R. (1985) Structure of problem behavior in adolescence and young adulthood. *Journal of Consulting and Clinical Psychology, 53,* 890–904

Dressler, W.W. (1988) Social consistency and psychological distress. *Journal of Health and Social Behavior, 29,* 79–91

Dryfoos, F.G. (1988) *Youth at risk. One in four in jeopardy.* Report submitted to the Carnegie Corporation. New York

Durkheim, E. (1951) *Suicide.* New York: Free Press (Original 1897)

Edelstein, B.A., & Michelson, L. (Eds.) (1986) *Handbook of prevention.* New York: Plenum

Elder, G.H. (Ed.) (1985) *Life course dynamics.* Ithaca: Cornell Univ. Press

Elias, N. (1987) *Die Gesellschaft der Individuen.* Frankfurt: Suhrkamp

Elliot, D.S., Huizinga, D., & Ageton, S.S. (1985) *Explaining delinquency and drug use.* Beverly Hills: Sage

Elliot, G.R., & Eisdorfer, C. (Eds.) (1982) *Stress and human health: Analysis and implications of research.* New York: Springer

Elliot, S.N., & Witt, J.C. (Eds.) (1986) *The delivery of psychological services in schools.* London: Erlbaum

Engel, G.L. (1962) *Psychological development in health and disease.* Philadelphia: Saunders

Engel, U., & Hurrelmann, K. (1988) *Psychosoziale Belastungen Jugendlicher.* Research paper, Universität Bielefeld

Engel, U., Nordlohne, E., Hurrelmann, K., & Holler, B. (1988) Educational career and substance use in adolescence. *European Journal of Psychology of Education, 11,* 365–374

Erben, R., Franzkowiak, P., & Wenzel, E. (1986) Die Ökologie des Körpers. In Wenzel, E. (Hg.): *Die Ökologie des Körpers.* Frankfurt: Suhrkamp, 13–120

Erikson, E.H. (1959) Growth and crisis of the healthy personality. *Psychological Issues, 1,* 50–100

Fagin, L. (1985) Stress and unemployment. *Stress and Medicine, 1,* 27–36

Faris, R.F.L., & Dunham, H.W. (1939) *Mental disorders in urban areas.* Chicago: University of Chicago Press

Farran, D.C., & McKinney, J.D. (Ed.) (1986) *Risk in intellectual and psychological development.* New York: Academic

Farran, D.C., & Cooper, D.H. (1986) Psychosocial risk: Which early experiences are important for whom? In Farran, D.C., & McKinney, J.D. (Eds.): *Risk in intellectual and psychosocial development.* New York: Academic

Farrington, D.P. Ohlin, L.E., & Wilson, J.Q. (1986) *Understanding and controlling crime.* New York: Springer

Featherman, D.L., & Lerner, R.M. (1985) Ontogenesis and sociogenesis: Problematics for theory and research about development and socialization across the life span. *American Sociological Review, 50,* 659–676

Felner, R.D., Jason, L.A., Mortisugu, J., & Farber, S.S. (Eds.) (1983) *Preventive psychology: Theory, research, and practice.* New York: Pergamon

Felton, B.J., Revenson, T.A., & Hinrichsen, G.A. (1984) Stress and coping in the explanation of psychological adjustment among chronically ill adults. *Social Science and Medicine, 18,* 889–898

Frankenburg, W.K., Emde, R.N., & Sullivan, J.W. (Eds.) (1985) *Early identification of children at risk.* New York: Plenum

Frankenhaeuser, M. (1981) Coping with stress at work. *International Journal of Health Services, 11,* 491–510

Franzkowiak, P. (1986) *Risikoverhalten und Gesundheitsbewußtsein bei Jugendlichen*. Berlin: Springer

Froland, C., Pancoast, D.L., Chapman, N.K., & Kimboko, P. (1981) *Helping networks and human services*. London: Falmer

Garbarino, J., Schellenbach, C.J., & Sebes, J.M. (1986) *Troubled youth, troubled families*. New York: Aldine de Gruyter

Garmezy, N., & Rutter, M. (Eds.) (1983) *Stress, coping, and development in children*. New York: Aldine de Gruyter

Gecas, V. (1981) Contexts of socialization. In Rosenberg, M., & Turner, R. (Eds.): *Social psychology. Psychosocial perspectives*. New York: Basic Books, 165–199

Gerhardt, U. (1979): Coping and social action. *Sociology of Health and Illness, 13*, 195–225

Goslin, D. (Ed.) (1969) *Handbook of socialization theory and research*. Chicago: Rand McNally

Gottlieb, B.H. (1981) *Social networks and social support*. Beverly Hills: Sage

Gottlieb, B.H. (Ed.) (1983) *Social support strategies*. Beverly Hills: Sage

Gove, W., & Tudor, J. (1973) Adult sex roles and mental illness. *American Journal of Sociology, 78*, 812–835

Gove, W.R. (1985) The effect of age and gender on deviant behavior: A biopsychological perspective. In Rossi, A.S. (Ed.): *Gender and the life course*. New York: Aldine de Gruyter, 115–144

Grant Commission (1987) *The forgotten half. Youth and America's future*. Report of the Commission on work, family, and citizenship.

Gurland, B.J. (1976) The comparative frequency of depression in various adult age groups. *Journal of Gerontology, 31*, 283–292

Haggerty, R.J. (1983) Epidemiology of childhood disease. In Mechanic, D. (Ed.): *Handbook of health, health care, and the health professions*. New York: Free Press, 101–119

Havighurst, R. (1956) *Developmental tasks and education*. New York: McKay

Hawton, K. (1986): *Suicide and attempted suicide among children and adolescents*. Beverly Hills: Sage

Heinz, W. (1985) Anstieg der Jugendkriminalität? In Rabe, H. (Ed.): *Jugend*. Konstanz: Universitätsverlag, 53–94

Heller, K., & Swindle, R.W. (1983) Social networks, perceived social support, and coping with stress. In Felner, R.D., Jason, L.A., Mortisugu, J., & Farber, S.S. (Eds.): *Preventive psychology*. New York: Pergamon, 87–103

Henry, I.P. (1982) The relation of social to biological processes in disease. *Social Science and Medicine, 16*, 369–380

Hildebrandt, H. (1987) *Lust am Leben. Gesundheitsförderung mit Jugendlichen*. Frankfurt: Brandes & Aspel

Hirschi, T., & Gottfredson, M. (1983) Age and the explanation of crime. *American Journal of Sociology, 89*, 552–584

Hollingshead, A.B., & Redlich, F.C. (1958) *Social class and mental illness*. New York: Wiley

Holmes, T.H., & Rahe, R.H. (1967) The social readjustment rating scale. *Journal of Psychosomatic Research, 11*, 213–218

Horn, K., Beier, C., & Wolf, M. (1983) *Krankheit, Konflikt und soziale Kontrolle*. Opladen: Westdeutscher Verlag

Hotaling, G.T., Atwell, S.G., & Linsky, A.S. (1978) Adolescent life changes and illness. *Journal of Youth and Adolescence, 7*, 393–402

House, J.S. (1981a) *Work stress and social support*. Reading: Addison-Wesley

House, J.S. (1981b) Social structure and personality. In Rosenberg, M.M & Turner R.H. (Eds.): *Sociological perspectives in social psychology*. New York: Basic Books, 525–561

Hurrelmann, K. (1984a) Adjusting to an erosion of opportunities: The experience of West German youth. *Policy Studies, 5*, 43–65

Hurrelmann, K. (1984b) Societal and organizational factors of stress on students in school. *European Journal of Teacher Education, 7*, 181–190

Hurrelmann, K. (1987a) The limits and potential of social intervention in adolescence. In Hurrelmann, K., Kaufmann, F.X., & Lösel, F. (Eds.): *Social intervention: Potential and constraints*. Berlin: De Gruyter, 219–238

Hurrelmann, K. (1987b) The importance of school in the life course. *Journal of Adolescent Research, 2,* 111–121

Hurrelmann, K. (1988) *Social structure and personality development.* New York: Cambridge University Press

Hurrelmann, K., & Engel, U. (Eds.) (1989) *The social world of adolescents.* Berlin/New York: De Gruyter

Hurrelmann, K., & Ulich, D. (Hg.) (1980): *Handbuch der Sozialisationsforschung.* Weinheim: Beltz

Hurrelmann, K., Kaufmann, F.X., & Lösel, F. (Eds.) (1987) *Social intervention: Potential and constraints.* Berlin: De Gruyter

Hurrelmann, K., Engel, U., Holler, B., & Nordlohne, E. (1988) Failure in school, family conflicts, and psychosomatic disorders in adolescence. *Journal of Adolescence, 10,* 237–249

Jahoda, M., Lazarsfeld, P., & Zeisel, H. (1971) *Marienthal. The sociology of an unemployed community.* Chicago: Aldine

Jason, L.A., Durlak, J.A., & Holton-Walker, E. (1984) Prevention of child problems in the schools. In Roberts, M.C., & Peterson, L. (Eds.): *Prevention of problems in childhood.* New York: Wiley, 311–341

Jessor, R., & Jessor, L. (1977) *Problem behavior and psychosocial development.* New York: Academic

Johnson, J.H. (1986) *Life events as stressors in childhood and adolescence.* London: Sage

Johnson, R.J., & Kaplan, H.B. (1988) Gender, aggression, and mental health intervention during early adulthood. *Journal of Health and Social Behavior, 29,* 53–64

Johnston, L.D., O'Malley, P.M. & Bachman, J.G. (1986) *Drug use among American high school students, college students, and other young adults: National trends through 1985.* Washington: National Institute on Drug Abuse

Kagan, A.R., & Levi, L. (1975) Health and environment. Psychological stimuli: A review. In Levi, L. (Ed.): *Society, stress and disease.* London: Oxford University Press, 241–260

Kahn, R.L., & Antonucci, T.C. (1980) Convoys over the life course: Attachment, roles, and social support. In Baltes, P.B., & Brim, O. (Eds.): *Life span development and behavior. Vol. 3.* New York: Academic

Kandel, D.B. (1980) Drug and drinking behavior among youth. *Annual Review of Sociology, 6,* 235–285

Kandel, D.B., Kessler, R.C., & Margulies, R.Z. (1978) Antecedents of adolescent initiation into stages of drug use: A developmental analysis. In Kandel, D.B. (Ed.): *Longitudinal research on drug use: Empirical findings and methodological issues.* Washington: Hemisphere, 73–99

Kaplan, G.A. (1985) Psychosocial aspects of chronic illness. In Kaplan, R.M., & Criqui, M.H. (Eds.): *Behavioral epidemiology and disease prevention.* New York: Plenum

Kaplan, H.B. (Ed.) (1983) *Psychosocial stress: Trends in theory and research.* New York: Academic

Kasl, S.V. (1979) Mental health and the work environment. *Journal of Occupational Medicine, 15,* 509–518

Kasl, S.V., Gore, S., & Cobb, S. (1975) The experience of losing a job: Reported changes in health, symptoms and illness behavior. *Psychosomatic Medicine, 37,* 106–122

Katschnig, H. (Ed.) (1981) *Sozialer Streß und psychische Erkrankung.* München: Urban und Schwarzenberg

Kaufmann, F.-X. (1980) Elemente einer soziologischen Theorie sozialpolitischer Intervention. In Kaufmann, F.-X. (Hg.): *Staatliche Sozialpolitik und Familie.* München: Oldenbourg, 49–86

Kaufmann, F.-X., Herlth, A., & Strohmeier, K.P. (1980) *Sozialpolitik und familiale Sozialisation. Zur Wirkungsweise öffentlicher Sozialleistungen.* Stuttgart: Kohlhammer

Kessler, R.C., & Cleary P.D. (1980) Social class and psychological distress. *American Sociological Review, 45,* 463–478

Kessler, R.C., & McLeod, J.D. (1984) Sex differences in vulnerability to undesirable life events. *American Sociological Review, 49,* 620–631

Kessler, R.C., & McLeod, J.D. (1985) Social support and mental health in community samples. In Cohen, S., & Syme, S.L. (Eds.): *Social support and health.* New York: Academic

Kessler, R.C., Price, R.H., & Wortman, C.B. (1985) Social factors in psychopathology: Stress, social support and coping processes. *Annual Review of Psychology, 3,* 531–572

Keupp, L. (1982) Zur Problematik der weiblichen Delinquenz. *Monatsschrift für Kriminologie und Strafrechtsreform, 65,* 219–229

Keupp, H., & Röhrle, B. (Ed.) (1987) *Soziale Netzwerke.* Frankfurt: Campus

Kobasa, S.C. (1979) Stressful life events, personality, and health. *Journal of Personality and Social Psychology, 37,* 1–11

Kohli, M. (Ed.) (1978) *Soziologie des Lebenslaufs.* Darmstadt: Luchterhand

Kohn, M.L., & Schooler, C. (Eds.) (1983) *Work and personality.* Norwood: Ablex

Kornhauser, A. (1965) *Mental health of the industrial worker.* New York: Wiley

Kosa, J., Zola, I.K., & Antonovsky, A. (Eds.) (1969) *Poverty and health.* Cambridge: Harvard University Press

Langner, T.S., & Michael, S.T. (1963) *Life stress and mental health.* New York: Free Press

Laosa, L.M., & Sigel, I.E. (Eds.) (1982) *Families as learning environments for children.* New York: Plenum

Lauth, G. (1983) *Verhaltensstörungen im Kindesalter.* Stuttgart: Kohlhammer

Lazarus, R.S., & Folkman, S. (1984) *Stress, appraisal and coping.* New York: Springer

Leavy, R.L. (1983) Social support and psychological disorder: A review. *Journal of Community Psychology, 11,* 3–21

Lerner, R.M. (1976) *Concepts and theories of human development.* Reading: Addison-Wesley

Lerner, R.M. (1982) Children and adolescents as producers of their own development. In *Developmental Review, 2, 4,* 342–370

Levi, L. (Ed.) (1971) *Society, stress and disease. Vol. 1.* The psychosocial environment and psychosomatic diseases. London: Oxford University Press

Levi, L. (Ed.) (1975) *Society, stress, and disease. Vol. 2.* New York: Oxford University Press

Levi, L. (1981) *Preventing work stress.* Reading: Addison-Wesley

Magnusson, D., & Allen, V.L. (Eds.) (1983): *Human development. An interactional perspective.* New York: Academic

Matarazzo, J.D., Weiss, S.M., Herd, J.A., Miller, N.E., & Weiss, S. (Eds.) (1984) *Behavioral health: A handbook of health enhancement and disease prevention.* New York: Wiley

Mattejat, F. (1985) *Familie und psychische Störungen.* Stuttgart: Enke

Mausner, J.S., & Kramer, S. (1985) *Epidemiology (2nd edition).* Philadelphia: Saunders

Mayer, K.U., & Müller, W. (1986) The state and the structure of the life course. In Soerensen, A.B., Weinert, F.E., & Sherrod, L.R. (Eds.): *Human development and the life course.* Hillsdale: Erlbaum, 217–245

McCubbins, H.I., Sussman, M.B., & Patterson, J.M. (Eds.) (1984) Social stress and the family. *Marriage and Family Review, 6, No 1/2.* New York: Haworth

Mechanic, D. (Ed.) (1982) *Symptoms, illness behavior and help-seeking.* New Brunswick: Rutgers University Press.

Mechanic, D., & Hansell, S. (1988) Adolescence competence, psychological well-being, and self-assessed physical health. *Journal of Health and Social Behavior, 28,* 364–374

Meyer, J.W. (1986) The self and the life course. In Soerensen, A.B., Weinert, F.E., & Sherrod, L.R. (Eds.): *Human development and the life course.* Hillsdale: Erlbaum, 217–245

Murphy, J.M., & Leighton, A.H. (Eds.) (1965) *Approaches to cross-cultural psychiatry.* Ithaca: Cornell University Press

Murphy, L.B., & Moriarty, A.E. (1976) *Vulnerability, coping and growth from infancy to adolescence.* New Haven: Yale University Press

Napp-Peters, A. (1985) *Ein-Elternteil-Familien.* Weinheim: Juventa

Navarro, V. (1976) *Medicine under capitalism.* New York: Prodist

Nestmann, F. (1988) *Die alltäglichen Helfer.* Berlin: De Gruyter

Newman, B.M., & Newman, P.R. (1975) *Development through life.* Homewood: Dorsey

Nitsch, J.R. (1981) Streßtheoretische Modellvorstellungen. In Nitsch, J.R. (Hg.): *Streß, Theorien, Untersuchungen, Maßnahmen.* Bern: Huber, 52–187

Oerter, R., & Montada, L. (Hg.) (1987) *Entwicklungspsychologie.* München: Psychologie Veralgsunion

Olk, T. (1989) *Die zwei Gesichter des Sozialstaates.* Berlin: De Gruyter

Oppolzer, A. (1986) *Wenn Du arm bist, mußt Du früher sterben. Arbeits- und Lebensbedingungen als Krankheitsfaktoren.* Hamburg: VSA Verlag

Osgood, D.W., Johnston, L.D., O'Malley, P.M., & Bachman, J.G. (1988) The generality of deviance in late adolescence and early adulthood. *American Sociological Review, 53,* 81–93

Parsons, T. (1951a) *The social system.* New York: Free Press

Parsons, T. (1951b) Illness and the role of the physician. *American Journal of Orthopsychiatry, 21,* 452–460

Pearlin, L. (1983) Role strain and personal stress. In Kaplan, H.B. (Ed.): *Psychosocial stress: Trends in theory and research.* New York: Academic 6–32

Pearlin, L. (1987) The stress process and strategies of intervention. In Hurrelmann, K., Kaufmann, F.X., & Lösel, F. (Eds.): *Social intervention: Potential and constraints.* Berlin: De Gruyter, 53–72

Pearlin, L., & Johnson, I. (1977) Marital status, life strains and depression. *American Sociological Review, 42,* 704–716

Pearlin, L., & Lieberman, M.A. (1979) Social sources of emotional distress. *Research in Community and Mental Health, 1,* 217–248

Pearlin, L., & Schooler, C. (1978) The structure of coping. *Journal of Health and Social Behavior, 19,* 2–21

Peck, M.L., Faberow, N.L., & Litman, R.E. (Eds.) (1987) *Youth suicide.* New York: Springer

Perry, C.L., & Jessor, R. (1985) The concept of health promotion and the prevention of adolescent drug abuse. *Health Education Quarterly, 12,* 169–184

Petermann, F., Noecker, M., & Bode, U. (1987) *Psychologie chronischer Krankheiten im Kindes- und Jugendalter.* München: Urban & Schwarzenberg

Petersen, A.C., & Ebata, A. (1987) Developmental transitions and adolescent problem behavior. In Hurrelmann, K., Kaufmann, F.X., & Lösel, F. (Eds.): *Social intervention: Potential and constraints.* Berlin: De Gruyter, 167–184

Petri, H. (1979) *Soziale Schicht und psychische Erkrankungen im Kindes- und Jugendalter.* Göttingen: Vandenhoeck u. Rupprecht

Pflanz, M. (1973) *Allgemeine Epidemiologie.* Stuttgart: Thieme

Rabkin, J.G., & Struening, E.L. (1976) Life events, stress, and illness. *Science, 194,* 1013–1020

Rickel, A.K., & LaRue, A. (1987) *Preventing maladjustment from infancy through adolescence.* Beverly Hills: Sage

Roberts, M.C., & Peterson, L. (Eds.) (1984) *Prevention of problems in childhood.* New York: Wiley

Rossi, A. (Ed.) (1985) *Gender and the life course.* New York: Aldine de Gruyter

Rumberger, R.W. (1987) High school dropouts. *Review of Educational Research, 57,* 101–121

Rutter, M. (1980) *Changing youth in a changing society.* Cambridge: Harvard University Press

Rutter, M., & Giller, H. (1983) *Juvenile delinquency.* Harmondsworth: Penguin

Sarason, I.G., Levine, H.M., Basham, R.B., & Sarason, B.R. (1983) Assessing social support: The social support questionnaire. *Journal of Personality and Social Psychology, 44,* 127–139

Schneewind, K.A., Beckmann, H., & Engfer, A. (1983) *Eltern und Kinder. Umwelteinflüsse auf das familiäre Verhalten.* Stuttgart: Kohlhammer

Schwarzer, R. (Hg.) (1985) *Stress and social support.* Berlin: Freie Universität

Schweinhart, L.J. & Weikart, D.P. (1987) Evidence of problem prevention by early childhood education. In Hurrelmann, K., Kaufmann, F.X., & Lösel, F. (Eds.): *Social intervention: Potential and constraints.* Berlin: De Gruyter, 87–104

Seeman, M., Seeman, T., & Sayles, M. (1985) Social networks and health status. A longitudinal study. *Social Psychology Quarterly, 48,* 237–248

Seidman, E. (Ed.) (1983) *Handbook of social intervention.* London: Sage

Selye, H. (1956) *The stress of life.* New York: McGraw-Hill

Siddique, C.M., & D'Arcy, C. (1984) Adolescence, stress, and psychological well-being. *Journal of Youth and Adolescence, 13,* 459–473

Siegel, L.J., & Senna, J.J. (1981) *Juvenile delinquency.* Sanct Paul: West Publisher

Silbereisen, R.K., Eyferth, K., & Rudinger, G. (Eds.) (1986) *Development as action in context.* Berlin: Springer

Simmons, R.G. (Ed.) (1981) *Research in community and mental health. Vol. 2.* Greenwich: JAI Press

Smelser, J.N., & Erikson, E.H. (Eds) (1980) *Themes of work and love in adulthood.* Cambridge: Harvard University Press

Snyder, C.R., & Ford, C.E. (Eds.) (1987) *Coping with negative life events.* New York: Plenum

Sobel, M.E. (1981) *Lifestyle and social structure. Concepts, definitions, analyses.* New York: Academic

Soerensen, A.B., Weinert, F.E., & Sherrod, L.R. (Eds.) (1986) *Human development and the life course.* London: Erlbaum

Srole, L., Langner, S.T., Michael, M.K., Opler, T.A., & Rennie, A.C. (1962) *Mental health in the metropolis. The Midtown Manhatten Study.* New York: McGraw-Hill

Strauss, A.L. (1975) *Chronic illness and the quality of life.* St. Louis: Mosby

Sussman, M.B., & Steinmetz, S.K. (Eds.) (1987) *Handbook of marriage and the family.* New York: Plenum

Thoits, P.A. (1983) Dimensions of life events that influence psychological distress: An evaluation and synthesis of the literature. In Kaplan, H.B. (Ed.): *Psychosocial stress: Trends in theory and research.* New York: Academic 33–103

Townsend, P., & Davidson, N. (Eds.) (1982) *Inequalities in health. The Black Report.* Harmondsworth: Penguin Books

Tuma, D.T., & Reif, F. (Eds.) (1980) *Problem solving in education.* Hillsdale: Erlbaum

Turner, R.J., & Noh, S. (1988) Physical disability and depression: A longitudinal analysis. *Journal of Health and Social Behavior, 29,* 23–37

Uexküll, T. von (1981) *Handbuch der psychosomatischen Medizin.* München: Urban und Schwarzenberg

Ulich, D. (1987) *Krise und Entwicklung.* München: Psychologie Verlagsunion

Waller, H. (1985) *Sozialmedizin.* Stuttgart: Kohlhammer

Wentworth, W.M. (1980) *Context and understanding. An inquiry into socialization theory.* New York: Elsevier

Wenzel, E. (Hg.) (1986) *Ökologie des Körpers.* Frankfurt: Suhrkamp

Werner, E., & Smith, R. (1982) *Vulnerable but invincible: A longitudinal study of resilient children and youth.* New York: McGraw-Hill

Wiley, J.A., & Camacho, T.C. (1980) Life-style and future health: Evidence from the Alameda County Study. *Preventive Medicine, 9,* 1–21

Wills, T.A. (1985) Stress, coping, and tobacco and alcohol use in early adolescence. In Shiffman, S., & Wills, T.A. (Eds.): *Coping and substance use.* New York: Academic, 67–93

Wirsching, M., & Stierlin, H. (1982) *Krankheit und Familie.* Stuttgart: Klett

World Health Organization (1946) *Constitution.* Geneva

Youniss, J. (1980) *Parents and peers in social development.* Chicago: The University of Chicago Press

Subject Index